# A SLIPPERY SLOPE

A middle-aged guy's bumpy run, from

**EARLY RETIREMENT** ...

to **SKI BUM** ...

to **SKI PATROLLER** ...

to **PHYSICIAN ASSISTANT!**

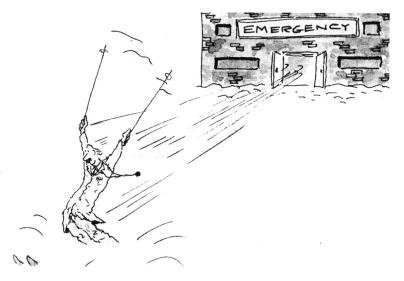

# Gerry Dougherty

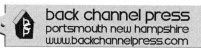
**back channel press**
portsmouth new hampshire
www.backchannelpress.com

# Table of Contents

## The Making of a Ski Patroller

## The Making of a Physician Assistant

# A Note About Editors

As sophisticated as I consider myself about the world in general, I found out I was pretty naive about the world of publishing. After I had finished writing part one of this book, I immediately set to getting it published. I sent several unedited copies to publishing houses in New York. I figured they were all sitting around dying to get the next great book idea. They are. This wasn't it. I never heard from them but I think I could hear the laughing all the way from New York.

I gave copies of it to a couple of folks on the ski patrol to read. They came back with similar sentiments. "Interesting pile of words you've got there. Why don't you find an editor." I had no idea how to do that.

Steve Barnes, on the patrol, suggested I contact a friend of his named Nancy Grossman. I did and that's how you come to be reading this.

Nancy and her husband John were immediately enthusiastic. They thought I had done something that was better than I thought it was.(If they didn't, they've managed to keep that from me for a fair amount of time.)

Nancy had a ready understanding about how sensitive we writers can be and that any little thing will send us into a snit. At the same time she immediately got what I was trying to do here and embellished it. Daily she would send me back little sections. It was amazing to me what a difference a word here or a changed phrase there could make. She rarely forced her opinion, but when she did I usually had to agree that her way sounded better. She also cured me of my habit of inserting a comma after every two words.

She is also responsible for part two of this whole thing. Part one had languished on my desk for a couple of years. One day I got an e-mail from her that asked, "So, are you ready to write the sequel?" I had already given up on part one ever going anywhere but before I knew it I had generated the second half of the book. It took some pushing and cajoling and the occasional stroking of my ego, but – here we sit.

The best thing about working with her was that she never lost sight of the fact that this was my book. She just polished and kept things pointed in the right direction.

For any of you who think you might be sitting on the next best seller...you could do worse than to run it by Nancy.

Give her a hello at backchannelpress.com. I won't be getting a finders fee, but you can consider my advice on this solid!

# Dedication

I've been told by my editor that I have to have a dedication page for this book. I hate dedications. People get all bleary eyed in attributing what is basically ink on paper to somebody in their lives.

It's been described to me as the same thing as naming a boat. Bad luck not to. My boat's not named. Here goes:

Marie Dececca: You won't get any monetary compensation for this, but thanks for the idea.

Tom Devane: You won't get any bucks out of this either but you planted the seed for a joy of a sport that became life long. Besides. You get to hang around with me on a regular basis and that can't be equated with a price.

My Dad: You were always there. I could not have completed all of this without your fiduciary and moral support. (Mostly fiduciary. There were weeks where I would have starved without a couple of bucks in an envelope.)

Christy Serra: You weren't involved in book one, but I doubt that I would have been able to get through all of the stuff in book two without you. We've had our ups and downs and I expect that we always will. I am so happy that you've decided to stay on the ride.

Enough?

# The Making of a Ski Patroller

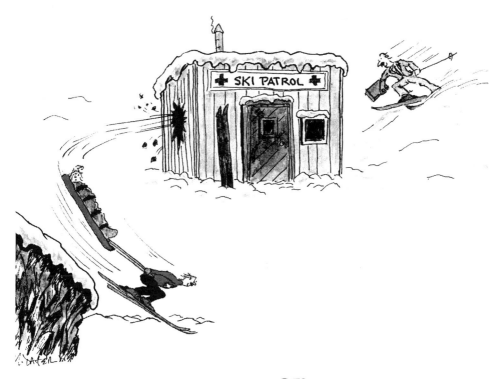

## or

### how I became a **sled dog** and **trauma junkie** in just a couple of months

# Introduction

Three months ago, I found myself hurtling down a trail on New Hampshire's Gunstock Mountain, toboggan in tow, bellowing for skiers to clear the way – a rookie ski patroller on my way to respond to only God knew what. I couldn't think about the frightening wailing I'd heard in the background when Karen radioed for help. I could only ski for all I was worth and hope I was equal to whatever I would find in the woods off the trail below me.

The same day one year earlier, I was settling comfortably into my new life as a 46-year-old, recently retired businessman turned ski bum. But the bum's life turned lonely and the offhand suggestion of a guy behind a deli counter last summer sent my life ricocheting off in a new direction.

\* \* \*

"Keep a diary." That was the advice my friend Marie Dececca gave me after I'd e-mailed her and told her that I'd started training to be a National Ski Patroller. Marie has some first aid training. She understood when I told her how involved the training was – and how surprised I was at that. She suggested that, if I made it, I might like to have something to read back through some day. I took her advice. I started to jot down a few observations every night when I got home from training.

I discovered immediately something I'd never anticipated – I was writing like I talk. I talk a lot. The diary started taking on a life, and form, of its own. It was never like this, years ago back in college. Back then, I was expected to write on demand, fulfilling uninteresting assignments that for whatever reason held no appeal for me. Words refused to flow.

After a while it occurred to me that I might just have a book here. Once that thought had surfaced and taken up a clamorous residence in my consciousness, I found myself consciously tailoring my writing to publication – I found myself picturing how every sentence would one day look on a printed page.

I didn't tell anyone I was writing a book. Upon soberer reflection, it seemed preposterous, especially in light of my subject matter. Who's going to be interested in a book about ski patrollers? A few ski bums, maybe a bunch of patrollers and other emergency providers? Of course it'd have to get published and into their hands. I didn't have a clue how that happens. Preposterous or not, though, I kept on writing. Mostly in longhand.

When ski season ended, I suddenly had a lot of time on my hands. I was not looking forward to transcribing my writing from my notebook into the computer, but one day I found myself sitting at the keyboard and I got to work. Before I knew it, I was spending lots of time, at all hours. I changed some things, wrote some more as memories came back to me.

Yesterday, I decided I was done. If you're reading this, then I guess I was successful in navigating the publishing process.

Once I started to write, my diary quickly turned into a labor of love. Love for a line of work that many people have never heard of, and love for the people who do it.

If you're a skier, you will probably never meet a ski patroller, at least under emergency circumstances. If you do, relax. You'll be in the hands of someone who is extremely well trained and dedicated to his calling.

If you meet one of these folks in the bar at the end of the day, have a good time. Ski patrollers can be a lively bunch.

If I make a couple of bucks off this, I won't be the unhappiest guy in New Hampshire, but that wasn't the reason for the project. My aim was to convey the day-to-day activity of a special group of people. I'm now on very familiar terms with most of the ones who work at Gunstock Mountain. People just like them work at every ski area in the world.

Whether you're a ski bum who gets in a few runs every day, or someone who heads south at the first sign of winter, I hope you enjoy what I've put together.

Marie – thanks for the idea.

Gerry Dougherty
Gilford, N.H.
May 18, 2002

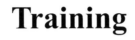

# Training

# September 2001

## Sept 4

Well. There I was, in the first aid room at the base of Gunstock Mountain, Gilford, New Hampshire. Of all places. And sweating. Not because of nerves – it was just plain hot. But the fact is, if you'd held a gun to my head, I couldn't tell you exactly what had inspired me to sign up for a course that's supposed to end up with me becoming a certified national ski patroller.

I mean, I know how I ended up there tonight, what had propelled me in this general direction. I'd stopped by one of those little country stores with a deli counter, to order a sandwich. The guy behind the counter was blathering on the way he always did as he threw together my standard fare. Ham and Swiss and "Hey, you ever give any thought to being a ski patroller. I'm gonna go through training, see if I got what it takes. Over at Gunstock. You interested? There's your lunch."

The deli guy was a ski lift attendant at Gunstock during the season. He'd seen me ski a couple of times. My style fit the criterion, he assured me. Looked like a cool job. Neither of us took into account screaming, mangled skiers. Neither of us thought, even remotely, about life or death decisions. We were both fairly sure that you got a free season's pass.

I guess I should mention that I'm 47 years of age – well into my 48th year on the planet, if you must know. At 4:59 on December 31, 2000, I retired from twenty-five years in the toy business, cheating my last employer out of one minute of my time and feeling not the least bit guilty about it – the way I saw it, the toy industry had cheated me out of twenty-five of my best years.

I hadn't retired impulsively. I'd planned it for many of those twenty-five years, salting away what finally added up to a respectable – and hopefully comfortable – sum. I've only done one impulsive thing in my life – sign up for ski patrol school.

The day after I retired I got up early and was standing at the front of the line at the lift ticket window at Gunstock when it opened for business. Not to buy a ticket for a day of skiing, no indeedy. "A season pass, please," I said to the woman inside the booth, savoring those four beautiful words.

I skied every single day last winter, whatever the weather, whatever my mood. And I did find myself getting decidedly moody. I was lonely, I finally noticed. Most of the time I had nobody to ski with. Everyone I knew was at work.

Ski season ended and I put my boat in the water. Gleefully, at first, I went out in it, day after day. And soon found that the same invasive loneliness had joined me on the lake. All my boating buddies were hard at work, too.

I attended a college reunion. As old friends volunteered what they were involved in, I discovered that my newly-minted status as 47-year-old ski and boat bum earned me few points and little respect. I didn't like the feeling.

Something had to give.

\* \* \*

When I was a freshman in college, my good friend Tom Devane asked me to come along on a ski weekend. I'd never skied in my life. My exposure to the sport was strictly Wide World of Sports and its weekly reminder of the "agony of defeat," timed neatly to coincide with some fool ski jumper's crash-and-burn. I assure you, trying the sport had never crossed my mind.

Me, I was into ice hockey, from the age of twelve. I loved the idea of skating on a frozen pond with no boundaries. The artistry of skating and stick handling brought with it an immediate sense of fulfillment. We had three ponds within walking distance of my house. I could be on them from late December well into March. I needed nothing more to improve my winters.

But Tom knew how to sum up skiing with a few key images. Girls. Warm fires. Girls looking for guys. Snow falling softly in the woods. Girls who like the thought of snow falling in the woods. Bartenders who liked the thought of snow falling in the woods. . He pushed all my buttons.

He was right. He hadn't mentioned the part about rocketing downhill, but I found that I liked that part, too.

I went straight from novice to fanatic. I wasn't very good, but I skied every time I could scrape together enough pocket change. I called my father and told him that somebody'd stolen my biology textbook. I needed money for another copy. Immediately. He sent it. A few weeks later, somebody stole my Spanish book. Another check arrived, enough to pay for a couple more lift tickets. American History finished off what was left of my credibility.

Enough time on the slopes and I started to develop some proficiency at the sport. I also started to notice the workings of the place. People were being paid to help me onto the lift. People worked all night, grooming the mountain and plowing the parking lot. People in uniform red jackets with crosses on their backs policed the slopes. I was never quite sure what their deal was. They represented authority, and they were around to promote safety. Beyond that, I really never gave them much of a thought.

* * *

And so I found myself looking around that underventilated, overheated room tonight, recognizing no one but the guy from the deli counter, starting on the road to what I guess I was hoping would be a new career. Me, Gerry Dougherty, certified ski patroller. I like the sound of that. On some level, I'd figured out that I needed a new career.

Chris Gamache, who conducted tonight's session, met the self-conscious stares of a dozen wide-eyed candidates with a look of seen-it-all bemusement. Thirty-something, thinning red hair, wire rim glasses, on first glance I pegged him as an accountant, or school teacher maybe – until I noticed that he's pretty solid. That started me thinking football coach, outdoorsman. Turns out he works for the state, in park management, environmental something or other. When he's not working his part-time winter job here as an EMT/patroller.

First mental adjustment: apparently this job isn't all skiing. We were all glancing nervously around the first aid room. Lining the walls were hospital gurneys and oxygen tanks. Splints. Rolled bandages. All manner of obscure medical paraphernalia. This being early September, it all looked pretty innocuous. Chris assured us this room will seem a lot livelier come early January. Gulp.

"So – why do you want to become a ski patroller," Chris asked each of us in turn. The answers were pretty much identical. "I love to ski. I'm a good skier. I can't get enough of it, any day, any weather. And I think I can deal with people who are injured." Chris told us that, in time, we'd get to do a little skiing.

"You'll find out real quick how you do with banged up skiers." A few of us laughed, nervously. "First things first. Make the check out for $115." The evening's session lasted maybe half an hour, tops.

Oh – have I mentioned that my latest girlfriend walked out on me last week?

## Sept 11

Class for tonight was cancelled. The world I thought I knew changed at 8:46 this morning. I've spent most of the day glued to my TV It is 4:47 p.m. as I write this, and I've watched those two buildings come down one too many times. And I've cried each time. Who could hate us so much? How could they do this to us?

# Sept 18

Straggling in for tonight's class, everyone was immediately drawn into the conversation about last week's horrific events in New York and Washington. Many of the patrollers are EMTs and paramedics and can't help but relate to what so many people had to go through. Several patrollers are making plans to go down to New York to provide relief for some of the crews. The discussion sucked the energy out of the room. Nevertheless, when a big, burly fellow with a shaved head stepped to the front of the room and clapped his hands to call us to order, we all quickly fell into seats and gave him our undivided attention. Frankly, I think we all found it a welcome relief to be able to focus the subject at hand.

Tonight we start our training for real. Our instructor is a guy named Steve Brennan. Very sure of himself for a guy who's only 26. Steve wants to know why we all want to do this. Clearly, we're a bunch of quick learners; this time most of us answer that we want to help injured people.

"Jeez, don't any of you like to ski?" Steve asks.

But most of the course tonight was taught by Sharon and Scott Davis. Sharon's an operating room technician. With hardly a hello, before we could even settle back in our chairs, she started right in, all business, briskly throwing around terms like "clavicle" (ah, yes, I think, collar bones) and "acromial processes," which I don't even have a clue how to spell. She led us through a whirlwind tour of the human body, a whole semester's worth of anatomy and physiology in about two hours flat. A subject I could have sworn I knew some about. By the time Sharon was finished, it was pretty clear that I barely know squat. I sat through the session groping myself, trying to identify all the parts she mentioned.

Sharon's husband Scott's a patroller up at Loon Mountain. (Loon likes to think of itself as New Hampshire's answer to Aspen.) Scott, a serious, methodical "Mr. Ranger Sir" kind of guy, clearly treats this profession with great respect. He assured us that any call can mean a life-threatening situation.

To illustrate his point, he brought up a well-publicized incident at Loon last year in which two experienced skiers went down a closed trail of sheer ice. One, supposedly a proficient skier, crashed into hazards and died. The second took off his skis and tried to climb down – only to slide to his death as well. I think Scott said he was a responder on that one. The moral of this story: never, *never* take off your skis, ice or no ice. At least you have an edge to work with.

He told us about another situation he was on where a skier took a bad fall and "smashed herself to smithereens" (a technical term, I assume). He thought she was dead for sure. Because of quick, competent action, she lived to ski another day. This I'm sure was meant to be inspirational. Me, I was thinking "May I never, *never* have to deal with anything like that.

Steve handed out our outdoor emergency manuals and the evening ended. Five pounds and easily an inch thick, the book in my hands looked like a cross between a high school biology text and something a first year med student would be finished with in a couple of weeks.

It's been 27 years since I last cracked a textbook – 28 since I actually paid attention to one. But who's counting...

# Sept 26

I came to class tonight having spent about three hours over the course of the past week perusing the text, in a general sort of way. Halfway through the week, I started to feel a bit overwhelmed. But I am determined to get all of this.

Tonight's class was all about initial assessment. A guy named Bob Ferris, who's both a patroller and a paramedic, conducted this session. Time to learn our ABCs all over again, he announced – rather gleefully, I thought. Nothing like first grade ABCs. Those were child's play. These ABCs are about life and death. A subject Bob seems to relish. His attention to graphic detail borders on the ghoulish.

A is for airway. Is it open? Can air get to the lungs? If not, the airway has to be opened by changing the angle of the jaw, or by inserting an artificial airway.

B is for breathing. Is the injured person breathing at a normal rate and in normal fashion? If not, breathing has to be assisted by artificial respiration. These days, that's mouth-to-mouth, with a twist. Because of AIDS and other communicable diseases, a barrier mask is used. We will all be provided with pocket masks. Steve stressed that you never give rescue breathing without the use of a barrier mask. Regardless, I can't help but feel that in a life or death situation, many rescue providers would go right for the nose or lips and start puffing.

C is for circulation. Are there signs of external bleeding. Do you suspect internal bleeding? Is there a pulse at the neck, wrist or groin?

It finally began to sink in that I may very well find myself responsible for some major issues with the mountain's patrons. All evening, as this realization sank in, we were also hearing what I'm sure was meant to be a reassuring counterpoint coming at us from various members of the teaching staff: we *will* get all of this, and we won't be put in the position of having to deal with something we aren't capable of. I have to say, I started the evening with a reasonably short mental list of situations I doubted I could deal with. By 10 p.m., this list reached well beyond the lower parking lot.

Bob Ferris apparently is famous for his cool. The more serious the injury or illness, the calmer, more matter-of-fact he becomes, I was told during break. It's said that you could drop right in front of him from a heart attack and elicit no visible reaction beyond his going into action to deal with the problem at hand. All business. Bob's parting thought for the evening: "Folks, you can fuss around all you want with a broken leg. If you miss anything serious with the ABCs, all you're going to have is a corpse with a nicely splinted leg. Read chapters 4, 5 and 6 for next time. Be ready for a pop quiz."

Isn't skiing fun?

## Sept 30

"Finding out what's wrong with someone is all about palpating," Sharon announced at the start of class tonight. "If you have any inhibitions about putting your hands on someone, or having hands put on you, then you're getting into the wrong business if you're considering ski patrolling." This elicited a few nervous giggles, then we got down to work.

Palpating: the squeezing, pressing and feeling of head, neck, chest, abdomen, extremities and back. You're looking for lumps, bumps, abnormalities, soft places that should be hard and/or hard places that should be soft. You're also trying to elicit pain responses from an injured person, to help you zero in on an injury. "The quickest way to find the site of damage is to get them to say ouch," Sharon told us. Several of us winced at the idea.

We spread some nice, thick blankets on the floor of the nice, warm lodge (hardly the conditions we'd be working under come ski season), then took turns finding pulses and palpating each other. For the most part, we didn't have the slightest clue what we're doing.

I knelt in front of fellow-candidate Diane Smith, who was playing the role of skier with a broken wrist. She's a good actress. I alternated between kind of patting and kind of pulling at the allegedly injured arm. Steve and Sharon observed my technique for a moment, then both barked out, "Hold it," almost in unison.

"Don't pat or tap," Sharon said, shaking her head. "You won't find anything that way." Steve knelt down and grabbed my arm at the shoulder and started firmly running his hands down my arm, lightening up slightly as he closed in on my wrist. He's obviously done this once or twice or maybe five thousand times before. He can probably do a full body assessment in about two minutes, he told me. "At this rate, it'd take you about an hour. You'd be dealing with a wrist fracture complicated by frost bite." I can't say I found Steve's confidence in my technique very comforting.

All this palpating feels totally foreign to me. It bears no relation to any other kind of touching one does naturally in life – hand-holding, hugging, amateur attempts at massage. Our instructors, knowing how unsure we were of ourselves, spent a lot of time with each of us. They also know there's a lot for us to master, and a limited time in which to learn it. The mountain opens in two months. They don't baby any of us. It's clear: we'll either get it or get run off.

# October 2001

### Oct 6

Driving to class tonight, I found myself thinking about how I'm attempting to get into a business dominated by young people. Like I said, I'm forty-seven years old. Many of my fellow candidates are half my age.

I've been married and divorced. I've had that successful, twenty-five year career in the toy business. I am somewhat financially independent (especially when you factor in the occasional hand-out from my dad, which he jokingly refers to as my "allowance"). Right now I'm just another doofus trying to keep straight on a whole bunch of procedures and protocol. It's humbling.

We candidates have spent enough time together now to be pretty comfortable with each other and our instructors. Recently, we've started having veteran patrollers show up and sit in the back of the room. They're here for a little refresher on their own technique, as well as to help out and give seminars on various specialties. I must say, it only adds to the pressure, having a new crop of strangers looking over our shoulders, observing our screw-ups. During breaks, though, they tend to be the center of attention, augmenting our textbook education with accounts of their most memorable exploits. Everyone has questions for them.

Tonight we were joined by a tall, rangy, good-looking guy in his thirties with a face that's got Irish written all over it. Everyone in the know seemed to defer to him, so I assumed he was a mucky-muck of some sort. He had several patches on his vest, none of which meant anything to me but seemed to be medically related. Turns out this was Pat McGonagle, supervisor for Safety Services at the mountain. He's also an intermediate EMT, which means, we were told, that he can offer more advanced courses of treatment, administer certain medications and start intravenous lines. Pat's got an easy-going way about him, and a pretty good sense of humor.

Tonight's subject was oxygen, the care and assembly of the equipment and administration to an individual.

Pat suggested we hold the oxygen canister like we'd hold an infant. "But – keep in mind that if you drop this infant, it could turn into something akin to a nuclear torpedo." I found that pretty funny. "I'm serious," he went on, straight-faced. "If you drop it and it hits the wrong way, it'll go right through that wall and out the one on the other side." Jeez. Everything round here has consequences.

None of us managing to blow up the lodge, we moved on to the various oxygen delivery devices. We also covered liters per minute to be delivered, and the amount of pure oxygen that is provided. Pat advised us that when administering oxygen, we should crank it up to the maximum amount that's recommended. "We can always buy more oxygen," he told us.

## Oct 9

Cuts and burns were on the agenda for tonight's class. And BSI – body substance isolation. That's how they refer to protecting yourself from the bodily fluids of another person in this great age of HIV and hepatitis. BSI, we were told, can't be stressed enough. In practical terms, this means putting on non-latex medical gloves, every time you approach someone. While we were learning, we didn't actually have to keep pulling on gloves, but we did have to call out that we were pretending to. You got yelled at if you didn't call out "BSI" as you came up on someone. This seemed kind of silly. On the mountain, I expect to approach a skier to answer his – or her, if my luck's running – question as to where to get a cheeseburger. However, I've come to trust that there's a reason behind everything we do.

Steve informed me tonight that my bandaging technique is terrible, and needs a *lot* of practice. I can tell he really likes me.

## Oct 16

On to fractures, sprains, dislocations and other discomforting boo-boos.

Tonight we learned that our job is not to diagnose a specific injury. Rather, we are "charged with the identification of a mechanism of injury," to put it in proper technical terms  Our job, then, is to "immobilize and stabilize the injured area." Only then do we get the injured party "the hell off the mountain" (*my* technical term for it), without making anything worse.

Two incidents were mentioned tonight that have come up before. They obviously made a heck of an impression on the patrollers involved. The first involved a young girl who was skiing for the first time. On her last run of the day, she fell and broke her femur (thigh bone). It was an open, or compound, fracture. The femur is the biggest bone in the body; you can imagine the force needed to break it – and the pain she was in. The bone had come through several layers of clothing. "It looked like a clenched fist sticking out of her ski pants," the first patroller on the scene told us. "She got the attention of almost every patroller on the mountain." They got her down in about eight minutes. The ambulance was already waiting for them at the bottom.

The other story had to do with an unfortunate fellow who took a tumble over the pointed end of his ski pole. The basket didn't hold. The pole went into his groin and came out through his upper left butt cheek. All I could think of was shish-ke-bab. As awful as his injury was, this was this guy's lucky day – the pole didn't hit any major internal organs. However, they did have to cut both ends of the pole off to get him through the doors of the ambulance. The part that was surgically removed hangs framed above the guy's fireplace today.

These incidents were discussed in almost reverent tones. Those relating these grim tales were entirely matter-of-fact about them. They never seemed to be grossed out. As for the candidates, my guess is we're all probably thinking the same thing: "Dear God, don't let me *ever* have to deal with anything even close to that."

Bob O'Connell, a patroller and the regional coordinator for the National Ski Patrol, helped out tonight teaching us the application of a Sager splint. The Sager is used to stabilize and apply mild traction to a broken femur. It looks like your typical medieval torture device.

The top of a Sager has a pad like the one on a crutch that fits into your armpit. On a Sager, this is fitted tightly into your groin. An adjustable metal bar runs from this to your foot. The splint is then strapped to your leg and ski boot. Tension is applied which creates traction. This not only stabilizes the leg, it also provides a level of comfort.

Bob can apply a Sager with his eyes closed. For us candidates, it looked like something that had dropped from outer space. We all gathered around to get a look at it, but nobody wanted to touch it. I can attest firsthand that when put on an uninjured leg, with tension applied, the feeling is nothing I could describe as comfortable.

Things have gotten decidedly more relaxed as we've all gotten to know each other. We can laugh over our feeble attempts and screw-ups. Our instructors laugh right along with us, but their laughter always ends up with, "Now do it again."

Bob also worked with us on applying slings and swaths to upper extremity injuries. He told me I could do with a little more practice. My current efforts, he thought, left my victims looking a bit too much like mummies. Clearly, I am really starting to impress these guys.

## Oct 23

Tonight was our midterm exam. Since the beginning of the course, I've spent an average of two hours a day studying. I want to be a ski patroller more than anything I've ever tried. Also, not having a real job, I certainly have the time to study – no excuses there. My almost 30-year-old credentials as a student should be considered questionable at best. I spent most of my four years of college in Providence, R.I., in a place called Brad's Bar and Grille. Back then, I was thrilled with a C.

I got a 96 on the midterm. I'm ticked off that it wasn't a 100. Still, it's the best grade I've had (without cheating) since the A+ I got in naptime back in kinder-garten.

# November 2001

## Nov 10

This weekend was about recertifying and refreshing the veteran patrollers. Up to now, the candidates have been the center of attention. This weekend, we were just there to serve as crash dummies for the veterans to practice on. It felt like having the upper classmen stroll in, after a week of freshman orientation.

Before we got started outside, a lot of general business was discussed. Several people read from this year's mountain guide. Someone noticed that every department and service the mountain provides has been mentioned – with the exception of Safety Services. What about us? Pat McGonagle explained it this way: "You want us in there? Okay. Next year we'll print it like this: 'Come on up. Have a nice lunch and a few drinks in our Powder Keg Lounge. When you go back out and have your serious wreck, our ski patrol's on the ready to scoop you right up.'" End of discussion.

We went outside and manned various areas which were being referred to today as "stations." It was cold and raw – it felt like snow. This wasn't the kind of day you wanted to spend lying on the ground, but that's where I spent most of it.

The observer at the first station was Craig Markert, a patroller and a doctor. "You have a fractured femur at mid-thigh," he informed me. "You're in great pain and slightly hypothermic." I could identify with the hypothermic part. I lay down on the ground and waited to be rescued.

Patroller Dave Farley, who'd introduced himself back in the lodge, came along and asked if I needed help. I dug deep, found the high school method actor within, and moaned that my left leg hurt like hell. He took off his pack and checked my breathing and my pulse. He asked if I'd hurt my head, neck or back. "Nope, just my leg," I told him through gritted teeth. He did a quick check from head to toe, then went for my left leg, while Doc Markert ticked off items on a checklist. Dave radioed that he needed a second responder with a Sager splint, oxygen and a toboggan. He then took hold of my left leg and pulled gently but steadily. It felt pretty good, without a real fracture.

Dave asked me if I used any medications. I figured a little levity might be in order. "Just Rogaine." Looking at my bald spot, he grunted, "Guess it doesn't work."

Mark Sugrue arrived and the two first simulated starting oxygen, then went to work on my leg with the Sager. As they started to push the pad into my groin, I mentioned delicately, "Guys, I dress to the left. Don't pinch anything important." Doc Markert leaned in and stage-whispered, "Don't flatter yourself."

All this was accomplished in about twelve minutes. Not all that long ago, it took me twelve minutes just to get the Sager out of the bag.

Doc Markert signed them off and they went on to the next station. For the remainder of the day, I was poked and prodded, had slings applied, was strapped to a backboard and was instructed to lie face down and pretend I wasn't breathing. It was a great learning experience to witness practical applications of the classroom scenarios we've been exposed to. It's also something *I'll* have to do in a couple of weeks in order to pass the class.

It was interesting to note that if veteran patrollers missed something, they were occasionally cut some slack. They were going through these exercises as much to shake off cobwebs as to take a test. They weren't under real pass-fail pressure, like we'll be when our turn comes.

It's a pity there weren't any Hollywood talent scouts around. I was good.

## Nov 11

Today was reserved for chair lift evacuation. I hadn't been looking forward to this – I was going to be one of the folks being evacuated. Frankly, I'm not real keen about getting down from anything more than three feet off the ground. However, I didn't have much choice in the matter.

We met at the Tiger Lift, which serves advanced skiing terrain. All the candidates and several veterans got onto chairs. The lift was run until we found ourselves a full forty feet off the ground. And then the lift came to an abrupt halt. We sat up there swinging in the wind, freezing our rear ends off. After a while (what seemed to me a *long* while), patrollers started to assemble under each chair.

Like everything else around here, this procedure is obviously well thought out and simpler than you might expect. Patrollers stood to each side of the chair. Another stood directly below it, coordinating between ground and chair. One of the patrollers to the side took a long coil of rope and threw it over the cable the chair's suspended from. This usually took several tries. The patroller on the other side grabbed the end of the rope. In unison, they used a lassoing/whipping motion to run a metal tube up the rope and over the cable. This piece protects the rope from friction damage, while also locking the whole shebang into place. A second rope with a wooden slat seat was then attached to all of this.

The slat seat was raised to the level of those of us being evacuated. Each of us in turn was instructed to pull it in and slide it under ourselves. Wearing a mountain climbing harness, one of the patrollers to the side proceeded to lower us down, one at a time. Another patroller kept a firm hold on the harness to prevent the first one from being lifted off the ground. All of this was being accomplished in three feet of rocks and overgrown grass. Four feet of snow and ice...hmmmm.

Doug Hamilton, overseeing the whole exercise, seemed to be having the most fun as he fired off jokes and generally made fun of everyone, dispelling the tedium while we all waited our turns. He also fired off suggestions like a machine gun. Once "rescued," each of us took our place working each of the ground positions.

A long day, but eventually everyone was down safely, trained or refreshed and back into the much-appreciated warmth of the lodge. Another year's recertification was over with.

## Nov 15

A ski town usually takes on an air of excitement about now. Natural snow has started to fall, or it's been cold enough for the snowmakers to crank up the guns and turn late fall into winter, on the mountain if nowhere else. Normally.

Not this year. Our weather's been coming in from Miami rather than Montreal. There's nothing more depressing than 65 degrees and bare slopes. I was ready to go back and break out my summer clothes when I heard the weather report this morning. The Weather Channel reporter looked positively proud of herself, rattling on about some freak high pressure system that's stalled over New England, with no end in sight. The golfers must love it. It looks like our traditional Thanksgiving opening is down the drain. Maybe I can be a ski patroller next year.

## Nov 20

Tonight was our last class before the final exam and technique certification. The topic was – childbirth.

I'd be willing to bet real money – a lot of it – that none of us will ever have to assist with a birth on any of our ski trails. I'd place a smaller bet that it won't happen in one of our lodges or the parking lot. Still, they assured us, it *could* happen. It's part of emergency responder certification.

Rae Mello, an emergency room nurse, led us through the material. As she got into some of the more – uh – difficult aspects of birth, Steve Brennan put his head down on the table he was sitting at and started to giggle – the kind of reaction you might expect from an embarrassed seventh grader. Rae paid him no mind, continuing through the subject matter. At the end of the lecture, Steve stood up and apologized. It seems he can deal with any type of traumatic event, but the mere mention of the subject of childbirth makes him nauseous and dizzy. I guess everyone has his Achilles heel.

The rest of the class was spent practicing backboarding. We've been doing this since our classes began. If you injure your head, neck or back, you'll end up strapped to a plastic backboard with a cervical collar around your neck. The idea is to accomplish this as quickly as possible while causing no movement to the injured party. It's challenging enough on the floor of the lodge. It's demanding beyond belief on a steep slope in deep snow.

Pat McGonagle brought along his eight-year-old son, Cameron, to serve as our injured party tonight. A levelheaded, composed little guy for his age, I remarked to Pat that Cameron seemed as knowledgeable about the procedures as we are. Pat explained that he's been practicing on Cameron since he was a baby. "Now all I have to do is say, 'Cameron, you've got a number twenty-two,' and he goes right into his dislocated shoulder posture."

Steve Brennan stood up at the end of class. "You're probably all going to make the cut," he announced. Several sighs of relief could be heard around the room. "I recommend you start buying your gear." He then went on to extol the virtues of Conterra's backpacks, for both their versatility and their many pockets and chambers. He also plugged Labonville's logger pants, which look like regular ski pants but are very rugged, very warm, and cost about half the price of regular ski wear. His enthusiasm leads me to believe that he's probably got financial arrangements with both companies.

# December 2001

## Dec 1

At 8:00 a.m. on this mild Saturday morning, we met for our final exam, which consisted of one hundred multiple-choice questions. A passing grade was 70. I got a 92. Steve Brennan graded each test in front of us.

I got a 91. I reviewed it quickly and found one Steve had missed. "What's the big deal over one point?" he asked me. "You passed." "It's real important to me," I assured him. "You probably wouldn't understand."

At 10:00 a.m., Steve said, "Okay, folks. The easy part's over. Let's get outside for the practical applications." Gulp! We've practiced all of this, over and over. We couldn't be more prepared. Now it was time for all the marbles. No one would be stepping in and setting you straight if you miss a step. Pass or fail. We filed out into the balmy December air.

I was paired with Craig Laurent, an immediate confidence-booster. Craig was a patroller several years ago. So much has changed in procedure and equipment that he had to take the class again to be hired.

Craig and I, it turned out, work well as a team. We moved from station to station where junior patrollers and people's kids were writhing for us in all manner of mock pain. We correctly assessed someone going into diabetic shock. We splinted a broken wrist and put a sling and swath on a dislocated shoulder. We splinted a blown-out knee and quickly reacted to someone lying face down, barely breathing. Each station was manned by a patroller with a checklist. The older ones weren't cutting us any slack. The younger ones occasionally gave us a wink and a nod on a minor misstep – but not if it pertained to a vital sign.

We finished up by applying a Sager to a broken femur and backboarding someone who was complaining of lower back pain. A few minutes later, Bob O'Connell gave us the news: we'd passed. We shook hands and patted each other on the back, two cool patrol school grads.

Eventually everyone straggled back into the lodge. Steve told us we were the first class he'd taught. "You guys have been a challenge," he said with a grin. "But I'll always have special feelings for each and every one of you."

We all jumped to our feet and gave him one resounding standing ovation as he passed out our diplomas. I don't think a piece of paper has ever meant so much to me.

"For those of you who are going to other mountains," Steve continued, "we wish you well. For those of you working at Gunstock, see you on opening day."

# On the Job

# December 2001

## Dec 19

Miracle of miracles: the mountain opened today. Gunstock's head snowmaker, who many consider to be the best in the state, has won a major battle with Mother Nature and gotten one trail open.

The paper this morning said, I believe, that we have three or four trails open. All ski areas tell fibs. Some tell outright lies. Most skiers know this and discount early and late season reports for that reason. I ask someone why we don't just state conditions as they are. "No one else will," I'm told, "so why should we?"

I walk into First Aid Base at 7:15 a.m., where Steve Brennan instructs me to go to the closet and pick out one of those coveted red jackets with the white crosses front and back. I find a brand new one that fits me perfectly. "Uh, not that one," Steve says. "How about this one?" He hands me one that's faded, its crosses more yellow than white. My "what gives?" look prompts him to explain. "You're going to cover up the crosses with candidate patches. I don't want to get pin holes in the new jackets. Great! We might as well be wearing fraternity pledge beanies. Everyone's going to know we're rookies.

But, as usual, there's a reason for this too. Passing the course is only about 20% of what's expected of us. We now have to prove that we can do everything on snow and in extreme conditions. We also have to learn all the aspects of the day-t-day routine.

Still, I'm wearing that red jacket. If I put my backpack on just right, it covers up most of the tell-tale candidate patches.

I introduce myself to Lee Bates. Lee has been a patroller for forty-five of his seventy years on this occasionally snow-covered earth. When he first started, nobody knew about oxygen cylinders, he tells me. If somebody got hurt badly enough, they'd be dumped onto a piece of plywood and carted down the mountain in something that looked like an old bathtub.

An engineer by training, Lee can come across as abrupt or curt. Some of the younger folks found him intimidating. I'd learned over the years, in other businesses, that if someone like Lee took an interest in you, you were going to learn a lot. "Let's get started on getting you certified," Lee starts right in. "Inventory the trauma pack."

A trauma pack is brought to the scene any time there's a moderate to serious accident on the mountain. Placed strategically around the mountain and inventoried each day, the trauma pack contains all sorts of medical goodies. I start by counting the different bandages and slings, checking each item off on a master checklist. I remove the oxygen cylinder and activate it to ensure that it's pressurized. I check off a variety of masks and tubing. I open the sleeve that contains nasal and oral airways, several of each in different sizes. Getting one of these inserted is not a pleasant experience. Then again, if you need one, you're probably not going to be conscious enough to care.

I finish by checking off several more gadgets. "Give me your check-off sheet," Lee says. He initials the box for morning base routine. I'm sure I must look quite proud of my performance. "Twenty-seven more boxes to initial," he states wryly.

The snow conditions are great on the one trail that's open. Since there are more patrollers on it than guests, Steve suggests, "Let's have some fun. Let's do some skiing exercises." He directs each of us to ski down while he and Lee observe our technique.

I think I'm a pretty good skier. I've skied for a long time. People who ski with me think I'm a pretty good skier. Steve calls me over and tells me why I'm not as good a skier as I think I am. "You look kind of pretty coming down," he says, "but your weight is too far back, your skis are too close together, and you're not finishing your turns."

"You just watched my second run of the year. Gimme a break!" I grouse. Steve tells Lee to work with me.

We take another run and Lee stays right behind me barking, "Stay forward, stay forward." He then yells for me to stop. As we both skid to a standstill, Lee says, "If you make one more turn that throws a rooster tail of snow in my face, you're going to have a ski pole planted you-know-where. Get on your edges and carve those turns to both sides."

A few more runs and Lee surprises me. "There you go," he says in an entirely different voice. "Now you're a completely different skier. Give me your check-off sheet." He initialed basic skiing. Only twenty-six more to go.

We spend the rest of the day doing all sorts of exercises. We snowplow from the top of the chair back down to the loading ramp. First one down's the loser. Non-stop snowplowing will turn your legs to rubber real quick, but this job calls for a lot of it. We ski with our boots totally unbuckled, making one quick turn after another. It's like trying to ski in slippers, but it forces us to get totally balanced. We also do a number of racing exercises. Much of this pertains to skills we need for the job. Some of it's ego. If you're going to patrol here, they want you to be a powerful skier, and to look good, too.

All in all, an exhausting but exhilarating day.

# Dec 26

The mountain now has runs open from top to bottom. While everyone else was eating Christmas dinner, the snowmakers were on the mountain lugging hoses and guns around. The snowmakers have a thankless job, and they're only too willing to explain this to anyone willing to listen. Most of their work gets done in the middle of the night. Not only is it physically impossible for them not to get soaked and frozen to the bone, the work can be hazardous in the extreme.

I don't think the snowmakers or grooming crews have much use for ski patrollers. We control the mountain – patrollers have the ultimate say as to what happens on the mountain. Regardless, groomers consider it *their* mountain. I get the impression they view patrollers as stuck-up pretty boys and girls. They're probably more than a little bit right, and they love the opportunity to stick it to "those idiots."

Now that the top is open, my second home for the next few months will be a small wooden cabin known as First Aid Top. Built of lumber that came right off Gunstock Mountain, it sports a handsome farmer's porch, but I doubt anyone gets much time to sit out there in a rocking chair. Inside it's furnished with a couple of couches, some picnic tables, a big wooden storage bin, all sorts of signs and rescue equipment, a big propane heater on the wall and a stove – but no refrigerator. Everyone's jackets, helmets and backpacks hang from pegs along one wall, all in a neat row, like stockings hung from the mantle on Christmas Eve. The dispatcher's desk sits in a corner by the window. My job today was to learn how to dispatch. We'll each take turns manning dispatch once a week.

Like police and fire departments, we're all tied into each other by radio. Active patrollers wear a harness that holds their communication lifeline, a Motorola two-way radio. The dispatcher records all radio communication and orchestrates patrol operations for the shift.

Each patroller has a "K" number for identification. I'm K-42. You might hear the following conversation: "K-11 told me he and K-24 are headin' to Patrick's Pub after work. You goin' with them?" It doesn't take long to learn the sixty or so K numbers and who they represent.

But very little gabbing goes on over the radios – they're a tool of the trade and most communication is economical and to the point. We use the customary "10-codes" that are standard to most emergency services. The most frequently used ones:

| | |
|---|---|
| 10-1 | I'm on scene |
| 10-2 | I'm out of service |
| 10-4 | I understand |
| 10-5 | Message received |
| 10-8 | I'm transporting an injured party |
| 10-27 | Call an ambulance |
| 10-50 | Injury accident |

Rather than saying "10-4" to acknowledge a message, we'll more often say "Copy." The terms "Roger" or "Roger Willco" are considered amateurish and thus frowned upon. I happen to like "Roger-Dodger" myself, but I keep it to a minimum.

We also have unofficial 10-codes. "Code Yellow" or "10-tinkle" – I have to pee.

An injured person is classified by status:

| | |
|---|---|
| Status 4 | Does not require further medical attention |
| Status 3 | Requires medical attention |
| Status 2 | Potentially life-threatening or -altering injury |
| Status 1 | About to die |

A typical series of communications might go like this:

*K-7*:    K-7 to First Aid Top.
*Dispatcher*: Go to Top.
*K-7*:    I am 10-1 at a 10-50, skier's right, Tiger Steeps. Stand by.
*Dispatcher*: Copy at 12:13 p.m.
*K-7*:    I have a forty-year-old female with a status-3 back injury and a previous history. I need a backboard, sled, trauma pack, and let's roll 10-27.
*Dispatcher*: Copy. K-28 is out the door at 12:15 p.m.

Translation: while out skiing, Karen Colclough comes across an accident on the right-hand side of Trigger, on a section known as the Steeps. She asks that dispatch stand by while she does a quick assessment of the injured person. As she performs her assessment, Audrey Beaulac yanks on her coat, helmet and backpack, ready to go if necessary.

Karen comes back with the information that the injured party is a forty-year-old woman with a suspected back injury and a history of previous injury. Karen wants an ambulance called.

Within two minutes of Karen's call, Audrey exits First Aid Top with the requested equipment. The injured woman will be strapped to a backboard and have oxygen administered. Audrey will then ski the toboggan down to First Aid Base, accompanied by Karen. The toboggan will be pushed up a ramp of groomed snow, through a trap door roughly the size of a large dog door, into First Aid Base and onto a carpeted platform. The two patrollers will shed their skis and hurry inside to assist the first aid attendant. The injured woman will be taken out of the toboggan and transferred to a gurney. A full body assessment can now be undertaken and all vital signs checked. Karen will get as much medical history as she can before the ambulance arrives.

My day as dispatcher started at 7:30 a.m. I got a snowmobile ride straight up the steepest trail to First Aid Top. I'm not all that enthusiastic about snowmobile rides on flat terrain under the best of circumstances. Add some slope and I can get downright nervous. This ride was not my idea of fun. Heidi Beaulac promised to go slow, but she said it with one of those suspicious-type gleams in her eye. We took off like the space shuttle. I somehow managed to get to the top without dropping my skis, lunch or radio.

The only skiing I'd be doing today was the run down when my shift was over. I walked into the building and took care of the first order of business: cranking the heat up to 75. The heater clattered and vibrated. I turned on the radio. "First Aid Top is now staffed and ready for business," I intoned in what I hoped was a fair approximation of a proper, seasoned – and glamorous – patrol dispatcher. "The temperature at this moment is 18 degrees, folks. The wind is blowing from the northwest at 10 miles per hour." I thought I sounded pretty darned good.

While I was involved with all this, the other patrollers were taking their first runs of the day. Each is responsible for the inspection and opening of a particular trail. If no hazards are encountered and if the condition of the snow and grooming are deemed to be in order, each will radio me that his or her trail is ready for the public.

When all the trails that serve a lift were skied and reports in, I called the operator and let him know he could open up. All of this was accomplished by the official opening time of 8:45 a.m. Each of the patrollers then caught the Summit lift, and were soon coming through the door. First Aid Top quickly takes on the feel of a locker room, but instead of padding around wrapped in towels, everyone clomps around in ponderous ski boots, heavy-duty waterproof pants and snug fleece vests.

We are a co-ed locker room. Because of this, most of us try to watch our language and subject matter. As in any locker room, there's some, shall we say, earthy conversation, perhaps a little more medically oriented than most locker room repartee but risqué nonetheless. The women on the crew either totally ignore it, or enthusiastically join right in. If anyone is offended by the direction that a conversation is taking, it's his or her responsibility to call out "red light," at which point the topic will be changed. We have very few red lights.

One of our female patrollers, who I'd assumed was purer than the new fallen snow, told me stories about her dog. She said that every night her dog gives her a big, wet kiss on the lips. I told her she shouldn't let the dog do that. She said it's a proven fact that dogs have cleaner mouths than humans. I told her that's an old wives' tale. "Your dog lays in the driveway and licks parts of herself that you wouldn't lick on yourself. Besides," I added, making a solemn attempt at seriousness, "you couldn't reach them anyway." She looked at me for a second and asked, puzzled, "How do you know I can't reach 'em?"

As the day went along, I got to feeling pretty comfortable with the radio and the lingo. I assume it's the way air traffic controllers and pilots feel after a while. I'm sort of like a controller; the patrollers are like pilots. Maybe not.

# Dec 27

I've been signed off for my stint dispatching yesterday. You have to dispatch during an accident to qualify. We had a minor one late in the day, enough to get another category taken care of.

Today I was patrolling. Candidates aren't allowed to go anywhere without a veteran patroller. No one has the confidence yet that we can handle a crisis on our own. My babysitter today was Curt Golder.

We took the early morning ride up the chairlift. The chair was covered with frost and snow. I mentioned that I was already freezing. "You should have worn your Hot Buns," Curt pointed out. Hot Buns are worn over your ski pants, covering your butt and upper legs with a layer of compressed foam rubber. They're held in place by a Velcro belt at your waist, as well as Velcro wrapping around your thighs. One more, very effective, layer between you and the elements. Curt had his on. I suggested he could have mentioned them while we were still in the locker room. "You rookies learn best from experience," he grinned.

At the top, the dispatcher told us to take a run down Flintlock. The trail offers a stunning panoramic view. We stopped and gave ourselves enough time to really take it in. "Make sure you do this every day, so you never take it for granted," Curt told me.

Gunstock overlooks Lake Winnipesauke. Winnipesauke is twenty-five miles long and dotted with hundreds of islands. The Ossipee mountain range rises from behind the lake, and the snow-capped giant, Mount Washington, juts up in the background.

At 6288 feet, Mount Washington is the Northeast's highest peak. As the world's mountains go, it's miniscule in altitude, of course; it's often referred to as the "rock pile." But due to its positioning relative to the jet stream, it has some of the wildest weather in the world. Winds of 100 mph are common. Sustained winds in excess of 200 mph have been recorded. The folks who staff the weather observatory up top supposedly have a cat that walks with a permanent list, from constantly having to lean into the wind.

People die on that mountain, on a regular basis. It's no place to take lightly. It's most famous attribute, bowl-shaped Tuckerman's Ravine with its legendary headwall, is credited as the birthplace of extreme skiing. No lifts service the Ravine – you hike up it and, the way I hear it, you're lucky to catch an edge a couple of times on the way down. I don't ski Tuckerman's. Never have, never will.

Today Mount Washington looked as stark as a moonscape, with the sun glistening brightly off its snow. I remarked to Curt that if Gunstock had a bit more altitude, we'd be prettier than Tahoe. "We're not that far off as it is," he replied as we took off.

We flew down the mountain at a much faster pace than we would had there been other skiers around. When we got back to the top, most of the other patrollers had arrived. People lolled around in various states of undress. Heidi Beaulac lay face down on one of the picnic tables, while her sister Audrey lay face up on the other one. People slouched on the couches with pants unzipped from ankle to hip and with legs hanging over the arm rests.

Ryan Mack was dispatching today. Looking out the window, he announced in a sing-song voice, "We have company." Everyone quickly came to attention, or at least a fairly close semblance of it, as a pretty young woman popped her head in the door and asked if she could come in and warm up. One of the guys actually started to tell her the warming hut was across the way. He was quickly drowned out by all the others telling her to come right in and join us. By the time she left a bit later, one of the guys had her phone number.

This job has definite possibilities.

# January 2002

## Jan 1

Not what they mean by a "Happy New Year." Just another workday. Last night I went to dinner at the home of my friends, the Hilsons. I told them about a lot of the stuff I've written so far. They seemed to enjoy the stories. Maybe there's a book here. We had a couple of beers and some great steaks. I was in bed by 9:15 p.m.

I'm told a lot of patrollers don't like to work on New Years Day. "Skiers come in hung over, get hurt and puke all over you," one of my colleagues informed me yesterday. Me, I had an uneventful day. Nobody so much as gagged within earshot.

## Jan 3

I was sitting in First Aid Top, staring at a picture of Jennifer Lopez in tight pants, when Curt Golder came over and passed his hand up and down in front of my eyes. "Are you signed off on knots?'

Oh, nuts. I shook my head no. "Let's have a go at it," Curt 'suggested' with a grin, pulling out some rope like a magician at a birthday party. I was no boy scout as a kid, and I'm no fisherman now. Just about the only interaction I have with knots these days is getting them out of my shoelaces. Which may be why I more than occasionally find my boat floating away from the dock, after I could swear I've tied it up securely.

Curt's both a boater *and* a fisherman. He was probably also a boy scout. He's the last guy I want to do this for. He was very patient with me, though, I have to give him that. He watched me do a truly competent square knot. Then he told me to produce a clove hitch. That took two tries. He ordered up a trucker's hitch. No sweat. Then he called for the dreaded bowlin – or bolin' or bowline. I groaned. However you spell it, it spells meltdown in my book. Or at least it did till Lee Bates took me though it, the other day.

"Way you do it, ya make yerself an inside loop in the rope. The end of the rope's yer rabbit. Rabbit comes up through the hole and goes 'round the tree. Then she comes back over the rope and back down into the hole. Grab her by the neck and pull tight." The rabbit survived. Curt signed me off anyway, though I gave him occasion to scratch his head a few times.

Ropes and knots are an important subject with patrollers. Rope's used for everything from marking hazards to both opening and closing trails. Nobody wants to be trying to undo someone else's impressionistic masterpiece on a cold night in January. All tie-offs need to be consistent.

Some of these folks can do more things with rope than the Boston Strangler. I'm afraid a lot of people will be able to identify my handiwork, at least for a little while longer.

# Jan 8

We've had several inches of snow in the past couple days. Unfortunately, it's come one inch at a time – better to get clobbered all at once and get it over with. I strolled into First Aid Top at 8:15 this morning.

One of the candidates, who shall remain nameless, was sprawled out on a couch. He's not yet of legal drinking age, but he managed to get loaded for the past three nights. His color was green. He hauled himself up and staggered outside for yet another round of dry heaves. Between trips, he told me he's never going to drink again. Having had some experience on this subject, I knew he'd be feeling well enough by 5:00 p.m. to break his vow. I related a story about Mike Royko, the renowned Chicago writer – and drinker – who once said words to the effect of, "If you think I'm drinking 'cause it's fun, then you probably aren't old enough to drink with me." The candidate, who didn't seem to get the point of the story, looked at me like I was speaking Martian.

# Jan 9

Today I hit the gym at 5:15 a.m. Dee Dee Goddard was there right beside me, pushing some weights around. Her husband Greg is general manager of Gunstock. I figured I better be measured in my conversation.

"How are the conditions?" she asked. "Pretty good," I answered, to which she responded, "Yeah, right. So, how do you like the job?" "It's great. "Yeah, right. How's Greg doing?" "He's a great manager." "Good answer."

We both went our separate ways to lift some more weights.

# Jan 10

Lee Bates informed me this morning that it was time to get signed off on basic toboggan work. The toboggan, or sled, is as crucial to patrollers as their radio. The candidates have all been practicing with one since the mountain opened.

A patroller's toboggan is about seven feet long, made of molded fiberglass, and weighs about sixty-five pounds empty. At first, we just pull empty sleds. The main idea is to pull a toboggan on a straight line. Injured people do *not* like to get bounced all the heck over the mountain.

I stepped between the long metal handles and clicked into my skis. Sled dog training 101 had begun.

I skied down the left side of Smith. Lee skied beside me at a leisurely pace. After about two hundred yards, he yelled for me to pull up. Turning my skis sideways into my standard hockey stop, the crossbar banged into my butt. "Look up the hill at your track," said Lee.

I looked up from whence I'd come. The trail I'd left looked for all the world like I'd been towing a writhing boa constrictor. Humbled, I asked Lee how to improve my technique. "Loosen your grip on the handles. Make more defined, quick turns and skids," he instructed me. I followed his suggestions the rest of the way down.

At the bottom, Lee said, "Well, looky there." I turned and looked back up the hill. The track was straight and true.

To load the sled onto the chairlift, I folded the handles back into it and clipped on a big metal bracket shaped like the letter C. I lugged the sled out onto the load ramp – a real trick with skis on – and the lift attendant slowed the chair down for me. As it came around, I lifted the C bracket up and slid it over the chair. Off we went.

Lee reminded me to keep a firm grip on the bracket. He worked with a patroller once who didn't, he told me. As part of standard procedure, patrollers announce on the radio that they're on the chairlift with a toboggan. A minute later, this guy's back on the radio announcing that he's still on the lift but his toboggan's MIA.

The penalty for dropping a toboggan off a chairlift is that you go back to skiing recreationally.

# Jan 11

Speaking of penalties, we have a system of fines for errors on the job. The whole thing is based on the honor system. Unless there's a witness, in which case you have no choice but to pay up. Errors and their penalties include, but are hardly limited to:

1. Fall while skiing. Put a dollar in the jar.
2. Fall where the whole world sees you. Put five bucks in the jar.
3. Go anywhere on the mountain without your backpack on. Buy a case of beer.
4. At day's end, we each ski down a trail after closing time, a chore referred to as 'sweeping.' We're looking for slow or injured skiers. At certain key areas, we have checkpoints with other patrollers. Miss a checkpoint. Buy a case of beer.
5. As I've said, drop a toboggan off the lift onto an open trail. Bye bye.
6. Have your candidate patches pulled because you've become a full-fledged patroller. Buy a case of beer.

I don't mind a buck every now and then, but these knotheads insist on premium beer.

# Jan 14

We had six inches of snow overnight. It looked like winter again this morning.

We were lounging at First Aid Top. Karen Colclough, who was dispatching, said, "Look alive. We have company."

A tall fellow poked his head in the door and said, "Anyone want to do me a favor?" All the veteran patrollers got busy with important tasks. Since I'd taken this job to serve the public, I of course leaped into action. "I can help you," I volunteered gallantly. My enthusiasm dropped a notch when I learned what he needed.

The fellow'd dropped his ski pole off the Summit lift, at tower 19. Oh, great. The steep hike down to it would be bad enough. Climbing back up through a couple feet of snow would be just like real work.

People drop all manner of paraphernalia off the lifts – sunglasses, hats, gloves, cell phones, skis, watches – how they loose watches I've never figured out, but they do. Heck – two or three *people* a year fall out of chair lifts. Typically, they're kids, and typically they don't get hurt in spite of 20 to 30 foot drops.

Clomping out of the building, I told him I'd meet him at the base of the chairlift. I stepped into my skis and took off down the trail that parallels the lift, but since the lift runs through the woods, I could only guess where tower 19 might be located. When I figured I was in pretty much the right neighborhood, I popped my skis off and started wading through the snow, aiming for the closest tower – which turned out to be tower 21.

I had no choice but to continue following the fall line down the mountain. I knew enough, however, not to hike down directly *under* the lift. Seems people on the chairs can't resist a moving target. I don't like to tattle, but snowboarders have been known to actually throw things at ski patrollers passing within range below them. I kept my distance.

Finally, I came upon the errant ski pole, grabbed it and started hiking back up to my skis, stopping every so often to huff and puff. Just in case anyone was watching, I pretended I'd stopped to take in the view. God forbid anyone should think I'm out of shape.

Even though we've gotten more snow, our weather's been outrageously mild. I'm starting to believe that global warming's for real.

It boggles our minds that the snowmakers have been able to open more trails, with nice conditions on them. This morning we opened Recoil, an advanced trail, which has always been my favorite trail on the mountain. Recoil's steep and long and undulates through the woods – good old-fashioned New England skiing. At the end of the day, I was assigned to sweep it.

Sweeping is performed in a nonstop snowplow position, cutting from side to side as we corral slow skiers along while simultaneously looking into the woods for anyone who might be there. At specific locations – those checkpoints I mentioned earlier – we stop and wait for other patrollers. We peer through the woods and click ski poles at each other, which translates as "so far, so good." It seems somewhat unnecessary since we all have radios. What can I say? Tradition. If you want to be super cool, you click poles behind your back. Also tradition.

About halfway down today, I missed a checkpoint. Steve Brennan immediately started shouting triumphantly through the woods, "That's a case! That's a case!"

When we got to Base, I found Steve to complain. "That's not fair. It's the first time I did that trail. I had no one to point out the checks." "That's no excuse. You had to point them all out on a trail map in order to get signed off," he replied without a trace of sympathy.

"Yeah, but they look different some times when you're out there," I protested. "Who signed you off on that anyway? he asked smugly. "You did," I smiled. "No way," he said. He stomped off to his office to consult the master sheet, returning with an appropriately sheepish expression on his face. "Okay. You buy half a case and I'll buy half a case."

Which isn't fair, if you ask me, but considering where we started, there seemed no sense in pushing it.
Oops. Am I whining? I occasionally whine. I know this about myself, and I try like the dickens to avoid it. Whenever I notice that I'm doing it, I'm quick to ask whoever's within hearing if I'm whining. More often than not, the answer's an unambiguous, "Yes." Sometimes, it's, "No way – you've got a point..."

In this instance, I sure wasn't about to give Steve the satisfaction of asking.

# Jan 15

I got signed off on toboggan pulling today. I'm now a certified sled dog. With Lee Bates observing, I pulled one of the other candidates from the top of the mountain to the base. I had to demonstrate that I could control the loaded sled and stop on command. I accomplished all this by sliding sideways on my skis, pushing and pulling on the handles and using the chain brake. (A chain, which sits between the handles, can be released to fall under the sled, providing control on even the steepest slope.)

After some hemming and hawing, Lee signed me off, figuring my technique's adequate enough that I won't lose a paying customer, at least. Incidentally, falling while pulling a sled also costs you a case of beer. I asked Lee what would happen if one were to lose a sled with a person in it. "Unthinkable," he said, "even if for some reason you should go head over heels. Probably best you impale yourself on one of those handles before you come to a stop."

At day's end, I was assigned to sweep Recoil again. I was so thrilled about hitting all those new checkpoints that when I got to the bottom, I enthusiastically announce on the radio, "Recoil's been swept. It is clear of skiers and closed for the evening." Silence. Karen Colclough came on the radio. "K-42, did you say that you're clear of Recoil?" She sounded somewhat gleeful, and I knew why immediately. Damn! I managed to miss a checkpoint on the other side that I'd hit at least a dozen times on other nights.

Steve Brennan came on the radio. "Uh, K-42, do you have stock in a beer company or something? You're on your way to a record for cases bought."

"D'oh," is all I can think to say, quoting the bard, Homer Simpson.

# Jan 16

As a candidate who's now an official sled dog, I'm qualified to pull an empty sled to an accident and give courtesy rides.

Courtesy rides are offered to guests who finds themselves on more challenging terrain than they'd bargained for. They're also offered to anyone who is just too tired to ski any further. Guests requiring multiple courtesy rides in any one day are considered a nuisance. They sometimes get a thrill ride designed to make them think about things.

Today I was called out to give a courtesy ride to a twelve-year-old boy. I was advised that it was his third ride of the day, and I was instructed to teach him a lesson. After loading him and his equipment into the sled, I set off on a course straight down the fall line. I had no intention of using the brake except in an absolute emergency. Cutting my skis back and forth, I intentionally threw snow in the boy's face. I found every bump I could. The toboggan went airborne, more than once.

At the bottom, I skidded to a hard and abrupt stop, and looked back, expecting to find the boy quivering, at the very least. Whimpering would be even better – though the effect I was really aiming for was out-and-out horror. What I found, rather, was a huge grin. "That was rad!" he enthused. I do *not* think he got the message.

# Jan 17

The mountain was pretty busy today. We got a couple of inches of snow last night. Today the sun was shining brightly and the temperature was right around freezing. Ideal. A lot of college kids still on their Christmas break were making the most of things before they roll into their next semester.

I was sitting on a couch at First Aid Top talking to Paul Kiely, a junior high school teacher who's maybe a little older than me. Paul usually patrols on the night shift, but works in a day whenever he's able. He's originally from New Jersey. After going to college at Dartmouth, he's basically never left New Hampshire.

Damon Hodgdon, one of our supervisors, fills in on a regular rotation when needed. Today he was dispatching. Damon grew up a tough kid, and was headed for trouble when he decided to put on the brakes and straighten up. When Damon gets bored, he throws knives around First Aid Top for fun.

As Paul and I talked, the phone rang. Damon had a matter-of-fact conversation with whoever was on the other end, hung up and appeared to go back to the paperwork he'd been preoccupied with since I arrived, so I figured nothing was going on. After a minute, he looked up and asked, "Who's up next?" Paul said he was. "We have a report of a young male with an arm injury at the intersection of Smith and Exit 20," Damon said. Paul grunted as he clamored off the couch and went for his coat and backpack.

Paul hurried out the door to grab his skis and poles off the rack, Damon turned to me. "Get ready in case Paul needs a sled," he told me, then leaned back in his chair and yawned.

My stomach tensed up. This might be my first chance to do what we candidates keep referring to, metaphorically, as 'the real deal.' I tried to fast-forward through every single thing I'd been taught in the couple of minutes that passed before Paul called in on the radio to say that he was on location. He had a nineteen-year-old snowboarder with an upper arm injury and was requesting a sled with trauma pack and a chaise lounge.

A ski patrol chaise lounge looks like a crude version of the classic summer backyard sunbather's recliner. It allows someone with an upper extremity injury to be positioned in the sled while sitting up, which is more comfortable than having to lay down under such circumstances.

Damon pointed at me, his fingers mimicking a gun, pulled the' trigger' and said, "You're on."

I grabbed a trauma pack and chaise lounge from the corner, hustled out the door and took my skis from the rack, then pulled a sled out from the group of them lined up next to the ski rack. It felt like it took forever to get my skis on, which I made up for by screaming down Trigger, yelling to people, "Make way! Sled on your left!" Startled skiers cleared to either side of the slope. I made a hard left onto Exit 20 and a hard right onto Smith, where I quickly came upon a group of people, skis off, huddled in a knot. Paul was kneeling in the midst of them, next to the young guy who was injured. I skidded the sled to a stop just above the circle of onlookers.

Very calmly, Paul said, "Gerry, why don't you get the sled and the chaise lounge opened up, and give me a couple of large slings." I jumped to follow his orders.

As soon as this was done, Paul directed me to play traffic cop. "Stand up there and make sure no one runs us over," he yelled over our injured skier's screams. Holy shit. Now I know what they mean by the expression 'blood-curdling.'

Through the screaming, Paul talked quietly to the kid, his manner soothing and composed. "I'm going to do something that's going to hurt for a second," he told him. I was wondering how much more this kid could stand. Paul rubbed the kid's neck reassuringly – then made a quick move, grabbing the arm and shoulder, appearing to affect a slight twist. Initially, I was thinking he was setting a break. As it turned out, he was returning the arm to its natural anatomical position. Clearly, I have lots to learn.

The young guy let out another serious yell, then dropped his head and started breathing deeply and slowly. It looked like he was feeling a bit more comfortable. Paul wrapped a couple of bandages tightly around him, immobilizing the injured arm against his ribs, then he turned back to me.

"Pull the sled down right next to us. We'll pick him up and get him situated," he said. This we managed to do causing only minor discomfort.

Directing me to pick up all the loose gear, Paul put on his skis and took the handles of the sled. He started off slowly, not wanting to cause any more joggling than he had to.

When we reached the base, we took the handles off the sled and pushed it through the trap door into the First Aid station. We jumped down from the wall and entered the room where Sharon Hannifan was waiting for us. She and Paul did a quick assessment. Sharon decided the injury was serious enough to warrant calling an ambulance. Paul took a medical history. I got a drink of water and sat, taking it all in.

After the ambulance arrived, Paul and I got on the lift back to the top. "Was that as serious as it seemed, Paul?" I asked. "That, Gerry, was about as bad a broken humerus as I've ever come across," he told me. "I could feel the bone pressing into his arm pit. That kid's going to need some serious surgery."

Note to self: Don't ever question someone else's pain. If they sound like they're hurting terribly, assume that they are hurting terribly.

\* \* \*

Gunstock offers night skiing. Several trails are flood-lit and open on most nights. The majority of our night skiers are families and teenagers, snowboarders for the most part.

Occasionally, you'll come across a guest who's operating under the influence of an "experience-enhancing substance." Sitting back up at First Aid Top, I asked Steve Brennan how you handle a belligerent guest. "The first thing you want to do is pop out of your skis," he told me. "Getting punched while you've got two boards attached to your feet puts you at a real disadvantage."

Pat McGonagle joined the discussion. "Try to reason with the person. If that doesn't work, do what I do. Yell JOOOOOOE." Joe Johnson, one of my fellow candidates, stands 6' 4" tall, weighs about 325, and skis like a heat-seeking missile. Think NFL nose tackle coming at you at mach speed. Joe has a calming effect on folks who might be otherwise inclined.

Pat concluded by saying that if the person doesn't appear to be in awe of Joe, "you should move away quickly and call the state police."

# Jan 18

Most of us make our own lunches every day and brown bag it to work. For the past eleven days, I've brought the same thing: ham and Swiss on a bulky roll, with potato chips and a Gatorade. Apparently, some people pay attention to this kind of stuff. "You ought to try going down some of the other aisles at the supermarket," Curt Golder told me yesterday. "They've got other kinds of food and things, you know."

Okay, change is good. For a change of pace, I decided to buy my lunch at the mountain today – though I do have to admit I was hoping they'd have ham and Swiss. Around noon, I announced that I was heading down to the lodge. Since I'm close to being signed off on all categories, it was decided that I could ski down by myself. A seventeen-year-old junior patroller named Ben King asked if he could come along. The other patrollers okayed the idea, "but don't get in any trouble," they counseled us.

Ben and I zoomed down Trigger and stopped at the Steeps. The conditions were nice, and there was a hint of snow in the air. We stood there for a couple of minutes, as much as anything to be seen by our guests – the public likes to see patrollers in evidence. I was waxing poetic about how lucky we are to be able to do this job when the radio crackled to life. "We have a report of an accident in the Trigger Steeps. Boy with a possible head injury."

"Hey, that's right below us," Ben said. I got on the radio and told them K-42 and K-107 would respond. Ten to one somebody up top was saying, "Oh, great. A possible head injury and those two goofs are the first to respond."

We each took a side of the trail. Halfway down, I came across two boys laying on their stomachs on the side of the trail, looking for all the world like they were just relaxing and watching traffic go by. I asked if somebody was hurt. The taller one points to his chunky friend and said, "Billy is."

I kicked out of my skis as Ben cut across the trail. Putting my hand on top of Billy's head, I asked him to take a deep breath. He did so with no problem. I asked him what had happened. He told me that he'd been snowboarding, went off the trail and hit his head on a tree limb. I asked if his head, neck or back were hurt. "Nope." I radioed to the top that we were on scene and to stand by.

I told Billy I was going to feel around a bit to make sure he was all right. He looked a bit dubious. I felt his head for lumps or indentations and looked for blood. Negative. I felt my way down his spine, checking for abnormalities. Negative. I opened his jacket and pressed on the four quadrants of his abdomen. There was no pain, but Bill was getting agitated – he wanted to get up and keep going. I told him not to move.

Meanwhile, First Aid Top was squawking for an update. I told them to stand by. Billy seemed to be fine, but he did tell me he'd hit his head, and agitation is one sign of a head injury. Just then Steve Brennan came on the radio and asked Billy's age.

"Twelve," I told him. Billy angrily informed me he was thirteen. "Backboard him," said Steve.

Two minutes later, Damon Hodgdon, Audrey Beaulac and Ian Hamilton showed up with a toboggan and backboard. Damon gave Billy a quick once-over and decided there was nothing wrong with him, but explained to Billy that standard procedure called for us to put a neck brace on him and strap him to a backboard. Billy told Damon where he could stick his [expletive deleted] backboard. Now both Billy and Damon were agitated. That was when Billy started running down the hill at a full gallop.

"Someone go get him," said Damon through clenched teeth. We all just stood there with our mouths agape, watching Billy disappear around a bend. "Okay, I guess I'll go get him," said Damon, and headed down the slope. We all followed in his wake.

As we were skiing, I asked Billy's friend if Billy had a problem controlling his temper. "Oh, yeah, big time," he told me. We pulled up just in time to hear Billy telling Damon off in language that would make a longshoreman proud.

Damon jabbed his finger at me, saying, "Escort him down. I'll go see if I can find out who he's with," and skied off in a decidedly foul temper.

We surrounded Billy who continued to march down the trail. I tried to talk to him in my most soothing manner. He bared his teeth like a ticked-off German shepherd, swearing continuously. "So Billy," said Ian Hamilton, "do you know any good jokes or something?" Billy replied to that overture by giving us the finger as he took off running again.

Reaching the bottom, I decided it was time to take charge of the situation. "Okay, my man," I told Billy, "now we're going to do things my way. We're going to go sit down, relax and wait for someone to come for you." At this, he took off running into the Stockade Lodge.

Ben and I ran after him. I guess I've watched too many police shows. Without thinking about it, I got on the radio and announced, "We are in pursuit of suspect at the Stockade Lodge."

We found Billy hiding around a corner. As soon as he saw us, he immediately started swearing and yelling. The lodge was jammed and this caused quite a stir. To my great relief, a chaperone from Billy's school arrived on the scene right about then. After a quick briefing on the situation, I was more than happy to turn Billy over to him.

Ben and I got on the chairlift to the top. He thought the whole incident alternated between humorous and exhilarating. I was beginning to wonder how all of this must have sounded on the radio, but I didn't have to wonder long. We were greeted with an entire spectrum of amused expressions when we got back to the top, having provided the entertainment for the week. Lee Bates suggested that in the future I should try to refrain from referring to our guests as 'suspects.'

# Jan 19

Saturday's usually a day off for me, but I'd asked Pat McGonagle if I could come in and work in the First Aid Room for the experience. He agreed that today would be a good day. I'd be able to observe Rae Mello, the trauma nurse, who'd be the attendant on duty. He reminded me that I'd be volunteering and that, of course, it would be a non-paid day. Of course.

I strolled in about 10:30 a.m., figuring things wouldn't probably start getting busy till around 2:00 p.m. It already looked like a war zone.

Rae was working on a young guy who'd walked in on his own, having fallen and hit his head. He knew where he was, but he wasn't altogether sure about what day or month it was. Ray strapped an oxygen mask on him.

Bob Ferris was holding the arm of a guy sitting on a gurney. Based on the grimace on the guy's face, I figured he'd probably dislocated a shoulder. Bob was trying to get the arm and shoulder into a sufficiently comfortable position that he'd be able to apply a sling and swath.

Pat McGonagle was strolling back and forth between a young woman laying on a gurney with an oxygen mask on, and a young girl sitting in a chair holding her elbow and forearm tightly to her chest. I asked him what's going on. "We pressed the 'Oh Shit' button about 9:30. It's been toboggans and ambulances ever since," he told me. "Take your coat off and dig in." So much for being the casual observer.

Some two minutes later, the trap door opened. Greg Gebhard backed in, pulling a sled, having already radioed ahead that he was bringing in an eleven-year-old boy complaining of back pain. Rae and I went over to the platform to assist Greg. Inside the toboggan was a little red-head. "Hi, guys. This is Kevin," Greg introduced us.

Greg had put Kevin on a backboard, applied a neck brace and had the boy wrapped up as tight as a burrito in a large sheet of canvas. "Kevin's initial complaint was back tenderness," Greg told us. "Now he's telling me his tummy hurts, upper left quadrant." Where your spleen resides.

Rae asked me to put on gloves and assist. She'd already gotten a blood pressure cuff on Kevin's right arm by the time I joined her. "Take his pulse," she directed me. It took me three nervous tries to find it. He was pumping a little fast. Rae thought his blood pressure was a little "soft" – another indication of a possible spleen injury.

"What happened?" I asked Kevin. He told us that he'd fallen and as he fell, his skis popped off. He bounced and landed on one of them, falling on his left side and back. He was still strapped to the backboard, but Rae managed to reach under and start pressing around on his back. When she got to the lower left side, Kevin winced.

"On a scale of one to ten," Rae asked the boy, "how much does that hurt?" About a three, Kevin decided. She asked how bad it hurt when he fell. About a six. Rae was no longer too concerned about his back. She came around, unzipped Kevin's jacket under the straps of the backboard and started pressing around the boy's abdomen. He was wincing visibly each time she pressed on either side of his upper abdomen.

Leaning to me, she said, "Have a feel." Gingerly, I reached inside Kevin's jacket and pressed the middle of his stomach, then the upper right and left sides. Kevin let out a little grunt. Rae asked me what I thought. "Unless Kevin here does a lot of sit ups, he seems a little firm," I answered. "He's also clearly tender in both upper quadrants."

"Yup," she agreed succinctly. She also didn't like his color, or the fact that he seemed a bit drowsy. "I'm drawing blood, starting an IV, and then Kevin, my man, you're going to the hospital," she informed her young patient, then went for supplies.

Pat, who'd finished up with what he was doing, now stood listening over my shoulder., then asked Kevin who he was here with. Kevin told Pat that his dad and sister were skiing some of the beginner trails. Pat went off to call an ambulance, and to have Kevin's father paged through Guest Services. Rae returned with a needle, an IV bag, a couple of vials and an alcohol swab.

Here's the deal, bud," Rae said to Kevin, in a voice that suggested he was an old pro at this kind of thing. "I'm going to give you a needle and draw some of your blood. Then I'm going to start a solution that's going to get some fluid running into you. Then you're going to take a ride in an ambulance."

"Is it going to hurt?" was Kevin's natural first question. "It might sting for a second," Rae answered, "but then you should feel much better." I'm not sure if Kevin believed Rae or not. I know I didn't. Every IV I've ever had burned like hell.

Rae gave Kevin's right hand a good wipe with the alcohol swab, then tapped a couple of times on a vein that was starting to bulge above his index finger. Kevin was already gritting his teeth. She popped the cap off the needle and quickly inserted it into the vein. Squeezing Kevin's knee for moral support, I forced myself to watch. She drew some blood, then handing me the vial, screwed another vial in place and drew more, then handed me that one too. Then she popped in the hose for the IV and hung the bag on a hook behind the gurney. Leaning over Kevin, she announced, "Done." Kevin smiled with obvious relief.

I asked what she thought was wrong with him. "Probably nothing," she answered. "But just in case there's spleen damage, this is what we do." She told me to write Kevin's name, the date and time on the vials, which I did. Ready to move on to the next problem at hand, she told me to keep an eye on Kevin.

We talked about sports and school. Kevin told me he really wanted to take off the neck brace. I assured him that for the moment it was going to have to stay put and that I knew it was uncomfortable, but that it was really for his own good. "Besides, before you know it, this'll be all over. I'll bet you're back here next weekend. Just don't come and see us in a toboggan again, okay?" Kevin smiled again.

Just then, his father walked in, grabbed Kevin's ski boot and gave it a little wiggle. As Kevin looked up and said, "Hi, Dad," his eyes begin to tear up a little. Most kids are very brave – until their parents show up. That's when the emotions come out.

I explained to Kevin's dad what the situation was and that as a precaution we were sending Kevin to the hospital. He told me he was willing to go along with whatever we suggested. The ambulance pulled in. Two EMTs came in the door with a gurney. It wasn't much past 11:00 a.m. and this was their seventh trip of the morning.

One of the EMTs turned to Pat and asked, "Can I at least go to the bathroom?" Pat replied, entirely matter-of-factly, "Take a dump on your own time. By the time you get this little guy to the hospital, we'll have another one waiting for you." Hiding one hand behind the other, the EMT gave Pat the finger. They both laughed – a little jocularity in the war zone.

Since Rae had started the IV, she had to go along in the ambulance. I watched through the door as she helped the crew load Kevin in the back. Then she climbed in after him and they were gone.

As I turned back to the room, the trap door popped open again. A sled was pushed through, then Bob O'Connell crawled in behind it. He stood up on the platform; I offered a hand so he could jump down. Pretending he was preparing to jump from a diving board, he grabbed my shoulder, dropping down while putting as much weight on me as he could. "You better knock off the goodies up top," I chided him. He winked.

Bob Ferris had been waiting for this one. Inside the toboggan was a blond girl, about twelve years old. It was her first time skiing and she'd injured her left tibia, above the top of her boot. She was clearly frightened and in pain, alternating between crying and going very quiet. Bob O'Connell undid the straps holding her in the sled and I started to pull back the canvas that was covering her. Bob Ferris wheeled a gurney over. A wooden and canvas "box splint" stabilized her leg from knee to ski boot.

Bob Ferris grabbed the girl under both arms, I put both my hands under her butt and Bob O'Connell gingerly held the injured leg. On the count of three, we picked her up out of the toboggan and slid her onto the gurney. She was heavier than she looked.

She started crying again. I came around and took her hand. "Where you from, gorgeous?" I asked. She giggled a little and answered, "Charlestown," though with her heavy Boston accent, it came out more like "Chahhleston." "Oh, a rough, tough city girl, eh?" She smiled through her tears.

Bob Ferris interrupted, "You two can flirt later." In spite of her obvious pain, the girl couldn't help giggling. "Gerry, give me a hand here," Bob continued, indicating with a nod of his head that he wanted to get her left ski boot off.

Taking a boot off someone with a leg injury can cause a lot of pain, but it frequently has to be done to get at the injury. Also, since we do it so often, it's felt that we're better at it than most hospital personnel. Placing my right hand under her leg at the injury sight and my left hand on top of her leg just below the knee, I held very firmly. Bob unbuckled and stretched the ski boot to the breaking point. He pulled it away from her heel very slowly, then slid it off while we both watched her face for signs that we might be hurting her. She winced once or twice, but finally the boot popped off.

Her big toe was sticking through the sock. "Hey," I said, "I've been looking for those socks. Where did you find them?" She giggled again. Bob unzipped the side of her ski pants and I rolled them very gingerly towards her knee. With this type of injury, this procedure can also be painful.

Bob started to work his way down her shin with both hands. He stopped about three inches above her ankle and, as he started to feel around in earnest, she started letting out little yelps. He worked down to her instep and felt for a pulse.

After a minute, he stepped back and motioned me over. "I'm sure she has a fractured tibia. She's in tremendous pain," he told me. Protocol called for an IV and some big-time pain medication. I went around to the right side of the gurney and taking her hand, asked her if she'd ever had an IV before. In a quivering voice she asked what I was coming to think of as the universal question: "Will it hurt?" I told her the truth: it would hurt for a little bit, but that Bob was going to give her something that would make her feel much better.

Bob was already kneeling at her left side, tapping and rubbing the inside of her left elbow. Pat came over, offering help if needed. "Get me a 19-gauge and a bag," Bob told him. Pat went to a toolbox that's usually padlocked. Fishing around, he pulled out a syringe, then went to the closet and retrieved a bag of saline solution. By the time he returned, Bob was swabbing the inside of the girl's elbow with alcohol. He quickly found the vein he was looking for.

The girl's eyes were glued on every move Bob made. I told her, "You have a choice, you know. You can watch him, or you can look at me. And as we both know," I said, doing my best Muhammad Ali impression, "Ah am very pretty to look at." This got a chuckle from a few people around the room. I was just beginning to wonder why I was wasting this tremendous talent, when this little girl turned away from Bob and locked eyes on me – and suddenly I knew exactly why I was here today, doing what I was doing.

Bob stuck her with the needle and she gritted her teeth. He drew back on the plunger to make sure he'd hit the vein squarely. A little trickle of blood came back, just what he was looking for. He cranked the hose from the IV bag into the needle, then came around and stood next to me. Producing another needle from his pocket, he rubbed her right hand with alcohol, looked at it for a second and took another jab. This needle had a pretty good dose of whatever pain medication he was authorized to deliver. "That's it. Fun's over," Bob informed her, upon which she relaxed visibly.

We heard the sound of the ambulance backing into its spot. We hadn't called them – they were here to drop Rae off. Pat went over to tell them we had another customer. Rae said, "Let me guess. You'd like me to accompany her to the hospital." "That's why we let you work here, Rae," Pat said. "You know the way."

The girl's aunt and cousin had arrived, looking for her. Perfect timing – they could all go to the hospital together. As we wheeled the gurney out, I looked down and asked, "How do you feel?" She looked up at me with a goofy expression. "I feel fab-u-lous." Even the EMTs, who've seen everything, laughed. The gurney was lifted into the ambulance and Rae climbed in after it.

I walked back in and sat down. This place was wild!

Just as this thought crossed my mind, the door opened up and a young woman stepped in. She was holding one wrist in the other hand. And she was very good looking. A really sharp-looking guy walked in behind her – this had to be either her boyfriend or her father, I figured. "I don't suppose you're going to let anyone else get near this one," Pat commented to me. "You've got that right," I said. "Well, then, go do something constructive."

I strolled over like the big-time patroller that I was and asked, "Can I help you?" She said, "I think my wrist is broken." Uh-oh. I ran to Pat. "Her wrist looks bad,"

I told him. "You better get over here." "Sorry, no can do. I have to look at a picture my daughter drew for me," he answered.

You just can't count on anyone anymore. I asked her if I could take a look at the wrist. She offered it up very slowly. Hand and wrist were headed at angles you don't see very often. She said again, "I think it's broken." After a very quick feel, I told her, "So do I," and asked her to hop up onto the nearest gurney.

It turned out this was her father she was with. On learning this significant fact, I vowed to myself that this lady was going to get world-class treatment.

I asked her to squeeze my hand, which she could barely do, but I didn't take it personally. I took her other hand and told her to squeeze. This one was strong. Assuring her that I'd be right back, I went for a sandwich baggie of ice and put it on her wrist, which caused her to suck air in audibly through her teeth.

"I'm so embarrassed," she confided in me. "I'm an expert skier. I can't believe I got hurt." I assured her that expert skiers had been leaving here all day in ambulances.

Her father started talking to her in terms that were coming to sound familiar to me these days. I asked him if he was in the medical profession. "Yes," he answered, "I'm a doctor." Oh, like I need that. Doctors think that because they've gone to school for years, they know more than ski patrollers who've taken a twelve-week course. I was amazed to find that this doctor deferred to my judgment.

I applied a cardboard splint to her wrist, then asked the doctor to hold it while I wrapped some tape around it. I then asked him to elevate the wrist while I applied some ice and checked her vital signs. I was sure he'd be as good as any nurse I'd ever worked with – had I ever worked with any nurses.

I gave father and daughter directions to the hospital, very sorry to see them go. Well, let's be honest. I was sorry to see *her* go.

The rest of the day was a total blur. I filled out medical forms. I ran to the door to assist people walking in with various injuries. I wrote stuff down. I took pulses. I gave hugs. I applied slings. I waited for the next sled to come through the trap door. At some point, Rae waved goodnight. I told her, "Thanks. All I got to observe was your ass climbing into the ambulance." She stuck her tongue out at me and off she went.

All of a sudden, I looked around and the room was empty and quiet. I looked up to see Pat standing against the wall with his arms crossed. He was smiling. "You did good, kid," he said. This from a guy at least twelve years younger than me.

We talked about some of the incidents that came up today. Pat would talk about medical stuff till the cows came home, or till his wife called *him* to come home, whichever happened first. I recounted the incident with the doctor and his daughter. Pat said, "A good doctor will defer to you. As far as they're concerned, they're in your territory. In fact, the last time that guy dealt with a wrist may very well have been in med school. He could be a kidney specialist, for all you know." I asked him what happens if you meet a not-so-good doctor. "That's where your winning smile and personality come into play," he told me.

"I don't know if you realize it," he went on, "but you have some of the trauma junkie in you. We all have a little bit of that going on. It's what makes us want to deal with people who are a total mess." Looking me over, he nodded like the old sage. "Yep. Trauma junkie. You might want to consider doing this full time." Well...maybe I'll look into it.

# Jan 21

We got about four inches of snow last night. This year, that qualifies as a big event. Normally, it takes about eight inches for anyone to even notice it's snowing. This is not shaping up to be any kind of a normal year. Last year, we got about 130 inches of snow, total – just a drop in the bucket by western standards, but a heck of a good year for us. This year we will be lucky to see 40 inches. Bless the guy who invented the snow gun.

Today dawned bright and sunny, with the temperature on its way into the mid-30s. It was going to be a busy day on the mountain.

I was at First Aid Top, sitting on a couch with Curt Golder. The other couch was jammed with more people than its seating capacity called for. An overstuffed relic of better days, this couch was referred to as the "life-sucking couch" – when you sat on it, it swallowed you up and sucked the life right out of you. Anyone who dropped onto it got an automatic nap. And needed help getting up and out of it.

With the morning sunlight streaming through the window and bathing the back of my head, I was having a hard time keeping my eyes open, regardless of which couch I was sitting on.

Sleeping on the job's officially forbidden. The official rule: it's perfectly fine to go to sleep, as long as you have your eyes open. Unofficially, an occasional catnap is sometimes justified, though only to be indulged when there are no supervisors around. At naptime, we cover for each other.

I was reading a very boring article on avalanche prevention. The next thing I knew, Curt was elbowing me in the ribs. "What'd ya do that for?" I asked, exasperated. "Your snoring was starting to make the building shake." Oh.

About 11:00 a.m., Steve Brennan called in. "K-2 to First Aid Top." Damon Hodgdon got on the radio. "Talk to me, Steve." Steve came back with, "I'm 10-1 at a 10-50, middle of Smith, at the first turn. I've got a 22-year-old female snowboarder. Status 2. I need a trauma pack and backboard sled, pronto. Roll 10-27. K-1 is also on scene." Damon responded, "Copy, at 11:04." At the same time, Sharon Hannifan at Base copied that she was calling an ambulance.

We'd all been quickly shaken out of our stupor. Status 2 is serious stuff. It just so happened that I was next in line to respond. Damon looked up at me and said, "Go! Go! Go!" I moved in three different directions at once. Coat, helmet, and Karen Colclough was holding my backpack up for me to slide my arms into. I rushed out the door, grabbed a backboard sled and pulled it into position, then ran back toward the door in time to catch the trauma pack Damon threw out to me, snatching it out of mid-air. I pulled my skis from the rack, snapped into the bindings and grabbed the handles of the sled, taking off skating to hastily build up speed. It was clear to skiers standing around that something was going on. They quickly cleared out of the way.

Since I was pulling an empty sled to an accident, it was appropriate to cover terrain as fast as I wanted. I decided to hustle. Cranking around a corner onto Flintlock, I was already at full speed. The sled fishtailed a bit behind me. Calling out warnings as I came up on groups of skiers, I imagined them spinning around in circles as I blew by them. Even though I was traveling at break-neck speed, I skated on my skis at every opportunity.

Coming around a corner onto Derringer, I slowed just a bit as I approached the merge with Smith. Once onto Smith, I put the brakes on. I certainly wouldn't want to go flying past the accident. Coming around the first turn, I came upon a snowmobile parked in the middle of the trail. People were gathered around, but I couldn't see Steve or Pat yet. Pulling right up to the scene, I finally found Steve kneeling at the injured girl's head, holding it stable. Pat was kneeling between her legs.

Steve and Pat had both been doing paper work in First Aid Base when the initial report was phoned in. They ran out, and spotting the accident as they looked up

Smith, they grabbed a snowmobile and hightailed it up the trail. Steve parked the snowmobile right above the girl so no curiosity seeker would accidentally run into her.

The young lady was out cold. They'd already inserted a nasal airway. When they'd arrived, she was breathing sporadically and making snoring sounds. Gee, I wasn't the only one snoring on the mountain . Now she was laying deathly still.

If Steve Brennan and Pat McGonagle weren't the two best first aid providers at Gunstock, they would certainly be on everyone's short list, though their styles differed markedly. It was an interesting contrast to observe.

Steve barked at me to get the oxygen tank out and activated. When I fumbled a bit, he growled at me. As he applied the oxygen mask, he barked at me again, this time to get the cervical collar and set it at medium neck size. In spite of his delivery, I was quite pleased that I accomplished this maneuver pretty quickly.

"You put it on," Steve said, still holding the victim's head. I knelt down on the snow, putting my head right next to hers, and gingerly slipped the collar under her neck and pulled it around. I positioned the chin piece and snapped it in place. Steve looked at me and said, "Well?" I looked back as if to say, "Well, what?" "Get the damn backboard out," he said through gritted teeth.

All the while, Pat, Gunstock's answer to Gary Cooper, was holding a one-sided conversation with the young woman in his most soothing manner. He pinched the inside of her thigh as hard as he could. She made no sound, but did manage to move her leg just a bit. Half talking to himself, Pat mumbled, "Well, that is not good."

I brought up the backboard and laid it on the snow so that it was up against her. Pat directed, "On the count of three, we turn her onto her left side. Gerry, you get her hip with your right hand and her back with your left." On the count, we turned her onto her side, a textbook move. Every part of her turned at the same time. I took my hand off her back and wedged the board under her, using my knees to make some minor adjustments. On a second count of three, we brought her down onto the board so that she was laying flat on her back.

Pat and I started to apply straps. The first two crossed over her upper body, followed by one across her hips and another across her legs. We buckled them all down, then finally secured a foam block on each side of her head.

I wasn't yet authorized to pull a sled with an injured person aboard, but both Pat and Steve had arrived by snowmobile and without skis. Steve tried to clip into mine, but they didn't fit. He didn't want to tow a seriously injured person down a slope behind the snowmobile. Without hesitation, he said, "You pull her. Take off." So I did, straight as an arrow. I avoided anything that even looked like a bump. I went like a bullet.

Later in the day, Steve said, "I didn't mean for you to go that fast with that sled. I could barely keep up with you on the snowmobile. The rule of thumb is, the more serious the injury, the more slowly you should be pulling the sled."

Chagrinned, I filed Steve's advice away. As it turned out, the young lady started coming around within a few minutes of arriving at Base. She wouldn't remember anything that had happened, but she'd definitely be getting headaches for a few days. Oxygen has a strong effect on people with head injuries, but it usually brings them around. It's considered to be a legal drug.

# Jan 22

Today's my birthday. I am now a 48-year-old rookie. In honor of this momentous event, I was assigned the morning snowmobile shift. Like dispatching, it's a job we each do once a week. I've quickly grown to despise "sno mo" duty.

The shift starts at 7:00 a.m. First you break the treads out of the ice, then start the machines up. They usually kick in with some conspicuous coughing and wheezing, after which the belching of smoke commences. Clearly, these contraptions don't like being left out all night. After checking over their general appearance and oil and gas gauges, you take each sno mo out for a quick excursion to wake it up.

By the time this much is done, the dispatcher is usually ready for a lift up to First Aid Top. Lee Bates is the only dispatcher who appreciates the slow, methodical pace at which I typically proceed. He's actually more afraid of snowmobiles than I am. His usual refrain of "uh – uh – uh" sets in when a sno mo hits 3 m.p.h.

The key for opening up First Aid Top is the sno mo chauffeur's responsibility. Forget the key and you're the one who gets to climb through the window, not the dispatcher.

On the way back down, the work begins in earnest. Under the seat, you're carrying an auger, a large portable drill. Its bit drills twelve-inch holes into snow and ice, their diameters designed to accommodate bamboo poles. And a lot of bamboo gets used on this mountain. Long shafts of red bamboo hold up signs, mark off hazards and stake up rope lines and fences.

Setting light-weight bamboo poles may not sound like much, but trust me, it's grueling work. The job requires plenty of strenuous up-hill climbing and plenty of wading into the woods in deep snow to dig out a rope or a sign. A lot of slipping and falling's involved. I have a huge purple bruise on my left hip from last week's outing. If you're not on your toes, you get to watch the auger go sliding down a trail. It travels faster than most skiers.

As a mountain that isn't off-the-charts challenging, Gunstock would be classified as a family resort. That and a very stringent insurance policy dictate the many fences and signs we utilize. I suspect we stake out more rope than any other ski area in New Hampshire, possibly more than all of them combined. And most of it gets taken down every night to prepare the trails for grooming, as part of the evening sweep – thus all the work setting it back up every morning.

Once the mountain closes for the evening, the groomers take over. The groomers rule the night, up there in their huge Piston Bully Snowcats. The cabs on these things contain all the comforts of home – big padded leather seats, great sound systems complete with CD players, you name it. Attached to the back of the cab is a mechanism similar to what you see on the Zamboni at the skating rink, which houses a huge grinding wheel and drags a giant piece of cloth the consistency of a fire hose.

The driver turns the heat up to 80 degrees, takes off his shirt, cranks up the tunes and heads up the mountain to start his night's work. He has no desire to stop and get out, should he come upon a sign or a rope. No, he'll be more inclined to run through any sign or rope that crosses his path – understandably so. Sometimes, however, a driver *will* get out. Which is why you'll sometimes notice the odd sign lodged some twenty feet up in a tree.

But far more often, all you find in the morning are beautifully groomed trails, the snow precision-packed, soft and ribboned with what looks like, and is called, corduroy. There is a remarkable exactitude to it, and it's a look early-bird skiers have come to expect when they arrive first thing in the morning. They rarely know, care or think about what goes into bringing conditions back to this point day after day all winter long.

On a good day, morning snowmobile duty will take the better part of two hours to accomplish. But with the auger and the snowmobile, the patroller with sno mo duty is a marked man. Every work order that comes up is going to be his.

By 10:30 a.m., I was sweating profusely and starting to get dehydrated. I was digging a rope line out of some ice when Steve Brennan pulled up on the other machine with a long list of additional projects to handle. Some of them were quite involved. "By the time the day's over, you're going to hate me," he said. "I already do," I assure him through clenched teeth. Neither of us smiled.

I finally got off the snowmobile at 2:45 p.m., and I was livid. I took the chair to First Aid Top, slammed the door open and threw my backpack across the room. Nobody said a word. They'd all been there. I just happen to be a bit more demonstrative in my frustration than most.

I stomped around a bit, then started yelling. "This job sucks. I joined the patrol to do first aid and to ski," I snarled. "Not to play the damned maintenance man for the mountain."

Very quietly, Karen Colclough volunteered, "Gerry, you're doing a great job."

I went off and sat by myself. When I'd calmed down a bit, I announced to no one in particular, "If you all come in some morning and the snowmobiles are on fire, you know who your prime suspect is." This generated a few smiles. "At the very least, I'm going to make those damn drill bits disappear," I added defiantly.

Lee Bates told a story that improved my mood, about a groomer at a very large mountain in northern New England. This guy was responsible for grooming some fifteen different trails every night. One night the heater in his SnowCat died just as he was starting his rounds. Being of tough New England stock, he didn't give it much thought – he figured he could make it through one night without heat. Wrong. He went into hypothermia, to the point of total confusion.

On arriving the next morning, his supervisor found one trail groomed as beauti-fully as he'd ever seen it. The other fourteen were untouched. And there was no sign of the groomer. The supervisor called the fellow's house. His wife an-swered. The supervisor asked for Ned

Ned's wife said, "He's in bed. Sound asleep. Is there a problem?"

The supervisor said, "Would you mind looking outside and see if anything looks unusual?" The wife came back on the phone and said, "My God, there's a SnowCat sitting on our front lawn." Ned had spent the entire night grooming the same trail, over and over, then had driven his Cat down the main road the two miles to his house. We all figured Ned's front lawn must have been the best-groomed lawn in New Hampshire that day.

I was so glad that today was just about over. It couldn't get much worse than this. Great birthday.

# January 23

You guessed it. Today was worse.

When I came in this morning, Steve Brennan asked me if I'd take a snowmobile ride up to the first aid shelter at Tiger Top. He needed a couple of signs we were storing up there. I told him I'd get right on it.

Snowmobile duty today belonged to Curt Golder. Since I now had a sno mo out, and since we had more than enough patrollers to open all the trails, I radioed Steve that I'd help Curt with morning duty. Steve had no problem with this, and Curt was absolutely thrilled. I've already described how I feel about this duty. I viewed this bit of volunteering of mine as a supreme sacrifice that I was doing for someone who's been as nice to me as anyone I've ever met.

However, within about two minutes, everyone but Curt seemed to have forgotten that I was just a volunteer. Steve called me with a job that was going to involve a steep climb up some icy terrain for some intricate (at least for me) rope work. I groaned and got on it.

The job took me much longer than it should have. At one point, Curt came along to thank me for helping him. We stopped to chat. Just then Steve came around the corner on another snowmobile.

"What are you doing?" he asked me. "I'm setting the line like you asked me to," I told him. "Not the way I want it done," he informed me. "Why don't you just get out of here. I'll do it myself," he fumed. Before I could respond, he continued, "Did you set the fence at the merge between Cannonball and Derringer?" I told him I had.

And then he got about as mad as I've ever seen him get. "That fence looks like shit," he yelled at me. "Do you have any idea what the hell you're doing?" Then he started carrying on about some other patrollers. He finished up with, "If you had any pride in what you're doing, this mountain wouldn't look like shit."

I was so mad I was ready to cry. Steve's bigger than I am, and tougher, but I was ready to start swinging. Instead, I walked away without a word and climbed on my snowmobile. I gunned it, then letting it rev, I turned and said, "I take a *lot* of pride in what I do." Slamming the snowmobile into gear, I sped away.

About an hour later, I was replacing bamboo on the Ramrod race course. It was a beautiful day. The snow was great. I thought to myself, you're one lucky guy to be working outside. I was as miserable as I've ever been in my life. If one more person said anything more inflammatory than "hello," I was going to quit.

I looked up to see Lee Bates skiing down towards me, carving big, lackadaisical, whistling-as-you-go kind of turns as he came. I was in such a foul mood that I didn't even feel like talking to him. He skidded to a stop beside me.

"Having a nice day, are you?" he asked. I suspect Curt may have told him of some of the morning's events.

"Lee, I've had it with this bullshit," I said. "I hate this fucking mountain and I hate this fucking job. I gotta tell you, at the end of the day, they can have this coat and their lousy seven bucks an hour and they can stick it." Which is about a full year's worth of swearing for me, though I may have done a little bit more.

Lee answered me very quietly. "I know you think Steve has it in for you, Gerry. I don't think he really does. Every now and then, everybody ends up in his gun sights. I know that at your age, and with the experience you've had in business, you feel like you've paid all the dues in life you should ever have to. However, no matter what your age is, you're a rookie here. I just think that sometimes a few folks around here forget that you're not a 20-year-old rookie."

He started to ski away, then stopped and turned back to me. "I don't blame you for wanting to quit. I sincerely hope you won't." He looked at me for a second, then skied away. We'll see.

## Jan 24

It rained all last night. When I got up to go to the gym at 5:15 a.m., a soaking, wind-swept rain was pelting down. I couldn't believe it. Things actually managed to get even worse yet. I was going to have to work in this crap.

The phone rang at about 6:25 a.m., while I was eating breakfast. It was Pat McGonagle. "We're not going to open today. I didn't want you to come in needlessly," he told me. Thank the Lord. I badly needed a day off.

## Jan 25

I woke up this morning feeling sore and nauseous. A flu's been going around, and it sure felt like it had found me. I called in and left a message on Pat's answering machine that I wouldn't be coming in. I slept for most of the day. My father drove up from the Boston area to take care of his little boy.

My paycheck for this week's not going to be worth the price of printing it.

# Jan 28

It's amazing what a few days off can do for a person, I thought to myself, waking up this morning to bright sunshine. I couldn't wait to get to the mountain and be with my buddies. I didn't even care that I had snowmobile duty this morning.

I was the first one in by about half an hour. As the rest of the patrollers filed in, they all asked if I was feeling better. "Fabulous," I told them, and I meant it.

Steve Brennan came in without so much as a good morning for anyone. He looked like he might have had himself a fairly lively weekend.

Heading straight for his office, he came back out a few minutes later to ask me, "What do you have left on your check off sheet?" Without having to look, I told him, "Trail closing for the early evening groom." This can't be accomplished without working an evening shift. "When are you scheduled to work a night?" he asked. Thursday, I told him.

"Give me your sign off sheet," he told me. I handed it to him. He proceeded to fold it up and pocket it. Then he said, "Give me your candidate patches." I grabbed my coat and started to unpin the patches. I wouldn't be quitting after all. It looked like I was being fired.

Steve took a hard look at me. "Predicated on you working this Thursday night, you are now a National Ski Patroller," he said.

It didn't sink in until everyone in the room started clapping and grabbing my hand. Steve stuck his hand out. I started to give him the patches. "Shake my hand first, ya dope," he said. I did. Then I asked if I could keep the patches. "Nope," he answered.

"First off, you've earned this. Secondly, we're severely short-staffed this week. Now you can pitch in on everything."
I was nothing short of thrilled. I departed First Aid Base walking on air. The cold seat of the snowmobile brought me back down to earth quick enough.

My first day as a National Ski Patroller was uneventful. At 4:15 we all participated in the sweep and declared the mountain closed. There's no night skiing on Monday nights. Once the parking lot was empty and we knew we were by ourselves, Steve locked the door and broke out the beer. I hadn't been doing much drinking recently. "Why don't you stay and have a couple of pops with us?" Steve suggested. "After all, you bought most of it."

I stayed. I was toasted for my accomplishment. I toasted back for the opportunity to have a second beer.

As we were chugging, Ryan Mack went to the VCR and popped in an extreme skiing tape. He and Dave Stiles were immediately glued to the TV. They viewed extreme skiing videos the same way I'd watch a tape of Cindy Crawford doing the dishes – presuming she was in her underwear.

Dave Stiles was in his early 20s, loud, brash, extremely confident and well on his way to becoming a paramedic at an early age. When I first met him, I remember thinking, "I'm not going to like this kid," but as I spent more time around him, I found it impossible *not* to like him. He reminds me of a bulldog puppy that just won't leave you alone. He's also enthusiastic and helpful. He has no problem being the butt of a joke – his philosophy seems to be that any attention is good attention.

Over the course of any week, Dave and Ryan take some horrific falls. Not because they're poor skiers – they're both tremendous skiers. They'll try any maneuver, on any type of terrain, under any conditions, and they're constantly egging each other on. The only thing they enjoy more than taking a bad "digger" is seeing the other take a worse one. If they weren't ski patrollers, they'd be getting thrown off the mountain on a regular basis. As they watched the incredible footage on the video, they were both back and forth at each other with "I could do that" and "like hell you could."

Completely mellowed out, I finally headed home and called my father, telling him I'd made the cut. He congratulated me. "You're too hard on yourself, Gerry. You need to relax and enjoy what you're doing. You're going to be good at it," he said to me.

I had to reflect, as I wrote this all in my diary tonight, that, as seriously as I was contemplating quitting, the act of keeping this diary may very well have kept me from it.

## Jan 29

I was on the early morning chair to the top, riding with Lee Bates. The sky was starting to look ominous. Snow was in the forecast and we were thrilled. As the chair crossed over Trigger, I looked up at the beautiful grooming. The only ski tracks on it were mine – I'd opened this trail about 20 minutes earlier.

I noted that at one point the uniformity of the corduroy started to go haywire and lead off towards the woods. "What do you think happened there?" I asked Lee.

He looked where I was pointing. "Oh, that's just Fish," he answered.

Fish is one of the better groomers at the mountain, Lee told me. On occasion a rabbit, porcupine or fisher cat will cross his path. Enduring middle-of-the-night boredom, Fish has apparently been known to take off after a critter in his SnowCat. About once a year there might be a little red splat at the end of his chase. Before any of you get all worked up, let me say: Fish loves animals. He just miscalculates every now and then.

A little further along, the lift started a steep climb up the side of a cliff. At the top was an area we call the "Smorgasboard." One of the lift attendants keeps the little plateau liberally sprinkled with bird seed and other assorted animal goodies. On a good day, it's standing room only for a crowd of birds, squirrels and chipmunks. Occasionally, you'll spot an owl sitting quietly off in a tree branch deciding who he wants for lunch.

A few days ago, just above the "Smorgasboard," I saw an animal scurrying across the snow that I'd never seen before. Covered with white fur except for a black stain on the end of its tail, it had a rubbery-looking pink face. As it burrowed under the snow, I could watch its progress as the snow undulated above it.

I got on the radio and told Curt Golder, our resident animal expert, what I'd seen. "That's an ermine," he informed me. "Member of the weasel family. They're tough little dudes." He asked if the ermine was swimming under the snow. I replied that it was. "He's looking for mice," he told me. You notice an awful lot of nature on the mountain, if you take the time to look around a bit.

Last year in late spring, Tiger had to be closed for most of a day. A black bear was lumbering around just off the trail, shaking off the effects of her long winter's nap. Her two cubs were wide awake. The braver of the pair would venture out into the trail, then dart back into the woods and up a tree. Some of the patrollers, determined to get a good look at them, ventured as close as they dared. The adult was still pretty groggy, but after all, mama bears command respect.

Around 11:00 a.m. it started to snow for real. I was on a chair with Scott Mooney. Both of us were quickly covered in snow. An EMT in town, Scott usually works a couple of nights a week as the base attendant. I'm more accustomed to seeing him pull an ambulance up to our door.

Scott said he was having a really hard time skiing in today's conditions. I looked down at his skis, which were easily ten years old and 225 centimeters long. I was surprised that he could even lift them. "Why don't you go see Nick Sandric, at Mountain Sports," I suggested. "He'll fix you up with some shaped skis." Scott asked, "Does he Pro Form?" "Absolutely," I told him.

Pro Forming is one of the great benefits of being a patroller. Since we're considered professional skiers, the industry has decided in its wisdom that we should be entitled to buy equipment at a discount – sometimes at a dramatic discount.

I dropped in to see Nick last Sunday. Looking up from behind the counter, he gave me a big smile, came around and we chatted for a while. He asked what I'd been doing. I told him I was now patrolling at Gunstock.

After a bit, Nick got down to business. "Can I sell you anything?" he asked. I told him I needed a pair of poles. He went and pulled out a pair of canary yellow racing poles. "How about these?" he said. Canary yellow's not really my color. "Just 'cause you're overstocked doesn't mean you should try unloading those things on me," I told him. He laughed. "This is a hot color," he insisted. "Get with it, man!" As I thought about it, I realized these poles would certainly be easy to identify. Lee Bates skis with pink poles for just that reason.

Just then I noticed a beautiful pair of Rossignol Power 9x's. Nick saw me looking at them. "Now that's a great ski," he said with genuine enthusiasm. "With your size and ability, they'll fly!" What the hell, I can always use another pair of skis. I asked, "You Pro Form, right?" He answered, "Of course."

I asked if he'd like to see my patroller ID "Of course not," he said, acting like I'd hurt his feelings. "I trust you." Then he casually asked me a couple of questions about another patroller. Once it was established that I clearly knew the guy he was talking about, Nick proceeded to trust me for real – and proceeded to suggest the top-of-the-line Rossignol binding to go with my great pair of skis as well. What could I say?

He went off the fill out the necessary paperwork. Ski companies closely monitor all Pro Form purchases – they'd prefer that you not buy on Pro Form for all of your friends. While he was writing up the purchase, I started looking at a pair of Atomic 9-20s, but pulled myself up short. No need to play Imelda Marcos in a shoe store.

Nick came back. "Skis, bindings, poles, six hundred sixty dollars," he said. Full retail would have been over thirteen hundred. Of course, any skier who pays full retail's not trying very hard. Still, I'd probably saved a couple hundred bucks over the usual decent deal. Nor do I think I'd put Nick into bankruptcy either.

"Come back in a few days and I'll have these all set up for you," he told me. "Why don't you take those ridiculous-looking poles with you now. They're turning off the customers." He gave me an exaggerated wink.

Today was my first opportunity to use my new skis. Nick hadn't steered me wrong. These babies are rockets.

At about 1:30 I was standing at the bottom of Tiger, leaning on my bright new ski poles, talking to one of my neighbors, when the radio scratched to life. Curt Golder came on. "We have a report of a possible 10-50 on Tiger. Is anyone in position to take it?"

I turned and peered through the swirling snow. About two-thirds of the way up, I could barely make out someone laying on the trail, and another person standing beside the fallen skier. I got on the radio. "Curt, I'm at the bottom of Tiger. It looks like that 10-50 is affirmative. It's skiers right, about a third of the way from the top." Curt replied, "Thank you. Lee's on the way."

I returned to my conversation with my neighbor. About a minute later, a woman skied up to me, asking, rather haughtily, if I was aware that there was an accident behind me. "Yes, ma'am," I replied, "we're aware of it. Someone's on the way. Thank you." Apparently my response wasn't good enough. Glaring at me, she said, "You're standing here doing nothing? Why don't you go and help?"

It's drilled into you from day one: patrollers are the ambassadors of the mountain. What I wanted to say to her is, "Why don't you mind your own damned business." Instead, I summoned my best smile. "Should I walk up? I might get there in an hour or so." She skied away in a huff.

She'd pissed me off. I told my neighbor, "Later," and skied over to catch the chair lift. As the chair came parallel to the scene, I yelled through the woods to get their attention, "Does anyone require help?" A woman shouted back, "He thinks he's sprained his ankle." I let her know that help was on the way. She shouted back, "Thank you."

I got on the radio. "K-42 to K-24." After a bit, Lee came back. "Go to 24." I could tell by the way he was breathing and the way his voice bobbled that he was cranking right along. I told him that the incident on Tiger appeared to be a lower leg injury. He responded, "10-4." I said no more. Lee would make an assessment when he got there.

Craig Laurent came on the radio to let Curt know he was at the top of Tiger. We keep sleds there. Curt came back, "K-44, please hold at Tiger top for K-24." Lee would let him know what kind of sled he wanted, if in fact one was needed at all.

I eventually got to the top, slid off the chair, looked over and waved to Craig through the swirling snow. I heard Lee on the radio, "That's a negative on Tiger." Evidently, the skier was feeling well enough to make it down on his own.

We can't force people to take a sled ride. Many of the scenes that we respond to end up being minor, or nothing at all. Like firemen, when the bell rings, we go.

Craig radioed Lee to wait for us, then we skied down to meet him. The three of us had a fun run down Tiger, thoroughly enjoying the conditions, then headed for the Summit chair, where we started yakking with Terry, the head lift attendant. He didn't necessarily share our enthusiasm for the conditions. For him, every day is a matter of basically standing around, stomping snow off his boots. Some days, of course, are worse than others, but for him the finest is no better than just O.K.

Lee, Craig and I took the chair back to First Aid Top. On the way up, I commented, "Ya know, this weather makes me kind of horny." Lee leaned across Craig and said, "Everything makes you kind of horny."

We got to the top and walked into the building, shaking snow off like a pack of dogs.

# Jan 30

I was dispatching. The mountain was very quiet. A lot of us in First Aid Top were getting caught up on our sleep. People! Don't you know that we have some fabulous conditions going for us here? Come up to our mountain and ski, for crying out loud!

About noontime, Damon Hodgdon walked through the door. "Hey, Bubble Head, wuzzup?" he asked me.

Before I started to patrol, I'd never worn a helmet in my life. I wasn't sure what to look for. A couple of weeks before the mountain opened, I went to the ski shop (where we're entitled to a 20% discount on all purchases). I must have been the first customer for the year. The guy who runs the shop just about leaped on my back, he was so excited.

I told him I needed a helmet. I said that safety, of course, was important but that I really wanted one that looked sharp. He rummaged around for a while, came up with an outsized purple one and plopped it on my head. Standing back, he surveyed the effect and announced, "That looks great. Fits like a glove, too."

After my discount, it only cost me $122.00. I couldn't wait to get home and try it on in front of the mirror.

Which is where I discovered that the guy had sold me a helmet that looked for all the world like a huge grape. Michael Dukakis lost a presidential election because of a tank helmet – and he looked a heck of a lot better in it than I did in this thing. After about two hours of adjustments, I got it to stop slipping sideways every time I moved my head.

The first day the mountain was open, I'd pulled it on with grim determination and yanked my goggles down over my eyes. I was ready to save the public.

Steve Brennan took one look and asked, "Where the hell did you find that helmet?" I pointed toward the ski shop. "How the hell much did you pay for it?" I told him. "You're supposed to get an employee discount," he said. I told him I'd gotten one. "Oh, man!" he said, loud, and walked away laughing.

Yellow ski poles notwithstanding, Nick Sandric would never have let me leave *his* store looking like that.

Soon after, complaining out loud to no one in particular that my helmet made me look like a damned bubble head, I learned a bitter lesson: I should never have made this remark within ear shot of Karen Colclough, for one. Now it's not uncommon to hear the radio squawk, "I'm on Gunsmoke. I need some bamboo. Have K-Bubble Head bring it."

Bad fashion aside, I believe that helmets should be mandatory. A lot of damage could be prevented if everybody wore them. Collisions between skiers, in particular, would probably be far less traumatic. New Hampshire proudly refers to itself as the "Live Free or Die" state. They don't make helmets mandatory for motorcyclists, much less for skiers. Lee Bates doesn't wear one. I wish he would. Everyone should.

# Jan 31

Tonight I worked the night shift. I'd been looking forward to this, thinking how I'd get to sleep in, get some errands done, and get to work with some other people for a change. However, today we got eight inches of snow. I found myself thinking, darn, I wish I were working with my pals.

I showed up for my shift at 3:30 p.m. Once again, I was the first one in, by a long shot. I chatted with Sharon Hannifan, who told me it had been another quiet day.

I listened to the chatter on the radio. It seemed strange not to be in the middle of it. For some reason, it felt like listening to total strangers, not the people I'd just about been living with for the past couple of months.

Around 3:45, I pulled my skis out of the closet and started the long walk over to the Tiger lift. When I got to the top, I took a hard right and skied up a little hill, popped out of my skis and walked into Tiger Top, headquarters for the night shift.

Turning up the heat, I proceeded through much the same routine I'd follow if it were morning at First Aid Top. I announced that Tiger Top was open and staffed for the evening. My call was acknowledged without much conversation. First Aid Top was busy orchestrating the sweep as the day crew started to close the top half of the mountain. Lonely and bored, I listened to my buddies conversing on the radio.

I looked up as Ed Consentino walked in. K-36. I realized I'd have to get on top of some new K-numbers.

Ed's the patroller that taught and certified me for CPR. An easy going guy who generally only speaks in bursts, he owns a True Value store over in the next town. He's also a paramedic. I'd peg him as being a little older than me. A lot of patrollers fit into the fifty to sixty age bracket, actually.

Ed works for Gunstock most evenings. I found myself wondering if he ever had time to get bored. I know he's content to spend most night shifts dispatching. He pretty much only goes out on bad wrecks, or when the action really picks up. I guess he gets his "trauma fix" on the paramedic side.

Craig Laurent was next in. Craig was working the swing shift, 10:00 a.m. to 6:00 p.m. Swing shift's designed so there's coverage on the mountain until all of the night crew gets in.

Craig's face was red from the cold. He'd skied down from First Aid Top carrying a trauma pack, which he threw on top of a table. He said he was pretty sure it hadn't gotten used at all today. I asked if he thought it needed to get inventoried. Before he could answer, Ed shot back that of course it should get looked at. Craig and I both went through it, annotating the check off sheet.

The radio crackled and a hoarse-sounding voice said, "K-52, Tower one, Tiger." Phil Tanner was on his way up. A little later in came Scott Taylor. After him, Scott Davis. Scott Mooney was in First Aid Base. We had the "Scott" market pretty much cornered tonight.

Last in the door were Kurt Webber and Dennis Cass, the night supervisor. Dennis is full-time National Guard during the day. He must get his fill of the military crap during the day – he's one relaxed supervisor at night.

He asked me if I play cribbage. I'm sure he was thinking, "Ah ha, a new mark." He looked disappointed when I told him no. He looked genuinely puzzled as he asked me, "How did you get on if you don't play cribbage?"

We have some serious cribbage junkies on this patrol. Lee Bates tried to teach me the game. I have to admit I didn't understand the scoring, and just plain didn't enjoy the game. I have some friends who may read this and nod their heads knowingly – in certain circles, I'm considered the worst whist player in North America.

"Congratulations on becoming a full patroller," Dennis said. "I understand that we have a technicality to clear up." We went outside and walked through the final exercise on my check off sheet. Satisfied, Dennis said, "I'll let Steve know you're all set." We went back inside.

Phil Tanner asked if he could ski. It wasn't his turn, but no one had any objections. Phil's "Regular Army" during the day. Given permission, he looked like the kid who'd been told he could take off his school uniform and put on his play clothes. He wasted no time getting out the door. Scott Taylor went with him.

The radio crackled to life. We heard, "This is First Aid Top signing off for Thursday evening, January 31, 2002. The temperature is 19 degrees, and the wind is five to ten miles an hour from the southwest. Conditions are currently light snow. Tiger Top, you have the communication." Ed copied First Aid Top's transmission. Responsibility for the mountain was now ours. Six trails were open for the evening.

Kurt Webber's an interesting guy. He's just retired as a professor at West Point and decided to settle here. He'll be teaching a computer course at a local junior college. Although he'd patrolled at a small mountain near West Point, Kurt was wearing candidate patches, which I'm sure thrilled him to no end.

A quiet and unassuming man, there's just the hint of a rugged physique under his fleece vest. There's more to Kurt Webber than meets the eye. He's been a member of some very elite special forces, which ones he won't say, but he did mention that going to work sometimes involved getting parachuted in behind enemy lines. He dropped hints of what he did, but I got the idea that a lot of it was still classified.

Back when I was in the toy business, I was sitting in a bar in Hong Kong one night with some people, including a friend of mine named Larry Snow. Larry excused himself for a minute and went to talk to a guy sitting in a dark corner, drinking by himself.

When he came back, I asked him, "Is that guy in the toy business?" Larry replied, "Yeah. You know him?" I told him I didn't. Larry told me, "That just happens to be as deadly a guy as you'll ever be around." I was dumbfounded. "That little mousy-looking guy?" I said, dubiously. "That little mousy-looking guy," Larry answered me, "could kill you with a rolled-up newspaper before you ever knew what hit you. He's trained to handle very special situations."

I said I didn't believe a word of it, but another of the folks we were with confirmed Larry's story. It's occurred to me that Kurt Webber might just know that little mousy-looking guy.

Things were pretty quiet, until Phil Tanner came on the radio. "I'm on the Tiger lift," he said, "and I'm looking down at eight snowboarders who are busy making themselves their own jump, in the Tiger Steeps. They even brought their own shovels."

Tiger Steeps was closed tonight. Not to mention that it's against mountain policy for any of our guests to build their own amusements on mountain property.

Dennis Cass looked at me. "Go handle that. If any of then gives you any crap, take their passes. Knock down the jump. Better yet, have them knock down the jump." "I'll take care of it," I told Dennis. "But he's coming with me," I added, indicating Kurt Webber with a thumb.

It took us about two minutes to get to the location, where we found a group of guys in their mid-teens, hard at work. Before I'd even come to a stop, I was talking to them. "Hold it, guys."

I clicked out of my skis as Kurt pulled up behind me. "Guys, you're on a closed trail. It's closed for a reason. Secondly, you're not allowed to make your own jumps."

One of them stopped digging and said, "Uh, you talkin' to us?" Kurt, doing an excellent Clint Eastwood, said evenly, "No. He was talking to me." I looked to see if he had one of those little black cigars sticking out of his face. He didn't.

The kids all started coming at us. They looked kind of menacing, like gang members in training in snowboard boots.

One of them announced, "This shitty little mountain doesn't have any jumps open yet. We're making our own." I replied, "This shitty little mountain will have the snowboard park open in a couple of days. Yours is now officially closed." Another kid said, "OK, but we'll each take one jump first." I said, "No. You won't." Somebody in the back of the pack imitated me in a sing-song voice. I suddenly understood why some people don't like teenagers.

"Listen," I said, "we're not trying to be hard-asses or ruin your fun. But if one more of you gives us any crap, we're taking all of your passes." At this, they immediately morphed from gang members into kids, all turning on the kid in the back, offering variations on "Ricky, why don't you just shut up," some versions more vulgar than others.

Kurt ordered them to get rid of the jump. Sullen, they returned to it and kicked it down. When they were done, I told them to line up. Kurt and I both produced our surgical shears. One of the bolder of them said, "Hey! I thought you weren't going to take our passes." I told him, "We aren't. We're cutting the edge off and writing our ID numbers on them." Standard procedure.

(The rest of standard procedure goes like this: If an offending skier's ticket gets pulled and he wants to get it back, he'll be invited to come spend a day shadowing the ski patrol, learn the Skier's Code and go through a mock trial intended to humble him into demonstrating an attitude that indicates he's ready to get it back.)

The biggest kid wanted to know what that meant. "That means that you've received a warning tonight. You get into another beef, the next patroller's going to throw you outta here."

Kurt and I started clipping the corners of their lift tickets and scrawling our K-numbers on them. The third kid in line practically whispered to me, "I've got a season's pass. Please don't cut it." I pushed him by. Quietly, he said, "Thanks, dude."

Things were finally straightened out. The kids started to put on their snow-boards. Kurt and I clipped into our skis. The kids went off ahead of us. We followed them for a distance; we wanted them to know that we were keeping an eye on them. It didn't take long before they were back to being loud and boisterous, yelling at each other and trying to knock each other down. They'll never know how lucky they were that there were no rolled-up newspapers around.

Later in the evening, Scott Davis asked me if I'd like to do some sled training. Scott, who lives in my neighborhood, usually works at Loon Mountain. Since we live only two miles from here, he often moonlights at Gunstock. Scott's considered to be a top-notch ski patroller. I jumped at the chance to do some practicing with him.

We went outside and he told me to grab a sled. It wasn't snowing as hard as it had been during the day. The flakes seemed to just hang in the air. The sleds were all turned upside down to keep them from filling up with snow. I took hold of one and started turning it over. It was already starting to freeze to the snow. I gave it a couple of shakes and it broke loose.

I headed down the trail with the empty sled. Scott alternated between skiing beside me and behind me, throwing out a couple of suggestions having to do with my hand placement. We came around a corner onto Tiger. Scott told me to hold up. I skidded to a stop and threw the rope that allows the chain brake to fall under the sled. "Hop in," he told me. He was going to show me his technique. In the process, he'd also get to show off.

I weigh about 220 pounds. With me in it, the sled weighed about 300 pounds. Scott lifted up on the handles and yanked on the chain rope. The chain slid out from under the sled and we started to slide along smoothly. I was enjoying the ride. Scott shouted things back over his shoulder, mostly technical, pertaining to his hands and momentum.

We came to a stop. Stepping out from between the handles and sliding to the left, Scott said, "Now I'm going to show you just how easy this is."

Putting one finger on the handle and allowing the sled to start moving again, he started skiing effortlessly in a "falling leaf" maneuver. Picture a leaf as it falls from a tree on a windless day. It rocks from side to side as it slowly falls. Scott was doing this on his skis, controlling the sled with one finger.

Have I mentioned that this is a very steep section of the trail? If I was pulling a loaded sled on this terrain, I'd have the chain down and I'd be making heavy-duty skids from side to side. I'd also be firmly situated between the handles.

O.K., I was impressed. We went a little further and he stopped, bored. "You bring it down the rest of the way," he said. "I'm going to do some skiing."

He started off quickly. Scott's a beautiful skier; he exudes power. He was making carved turns, sling-shotting out of each one with ever more speed. By the time he reached the bottom, he was at racing speed. I'd been skiing along leisurely with the sled, enjoying the show.

At the very bottom, he made a hard turn to the left, looking like he was planning on skiing uphill on Cannonball until his velocity slowed, at which point he'd turn and slowly slide back down. Cannonball was closed and in darkness – that's why he was headed that way.

However, I seriously doubt that Scott's plans included the rope that was stretched tightly across the bottom of Cannonball, about waist high. He spotted it a moment too late.

Trying to jump over it, his skis cracked together and flew off in different directions. His foot just barely hit the rope as he soared over it. That was enough to rotate him so he was now flying through the air backwards, looking like he was sitting down. If he had a newspaper in his hands, he'd look like he was sitting on the toilet. He flew past a lift tower and landed in a snow bank with a very audible, "Boof." Picking up the pace very quickly, I yelled, "Scott!" I was hoping I wouldn't have to put the sled into service.

Sliding to a stop, I yelled again, "Scott! Scott, are you all right?" He was still sitting, his ski cap pushed way back on his head. Broken in half, one side of his goggles was where it was supposed to be, over his left eye. The other side was lodged down below his chin.

Covered with snow, he seemed to be taking inventory. When he was satisfied that all of his parts were still attached, he got up rather gingerly. Then he started to giggle. And I started to roar with laughter. I'll never forget the sight of him soaring through the air backwards with this totally perplexed look on his face.

"The last time I took a digger like that," he said, "I had to go visit the surgeon." Flexing his right knee, he said, "Humpf. I guess he did a pretty good job. Still works."

I don't know if Scott put a dollar in the jar or not, but I'd gladly put several in for having had the great good fortune to witness his performance – if that were a rule.

The mountain was due to close in about twenty minutes. Dennis Cass asked me if I'd like to take a run with him. He hadn't gotten much skiing in tonight – he'd been stuck in a winning streak at cribbage.

As we went outside, I mentioned I'd noticed that I'm having a problem with my depth perception, not picking up the bumps or icy spots as well as I would during the day. "You get used to it after a while," Dennis assued me, "but it'll never be the same as in natural light."

"We'll ski along the side of the trail where snow's piled up," he said, then took off, me following behind. He skied in a style that was very popular during the 1970s and '80s, before the advent of shaped skis, making little turns punctuated with little hops in between. I started to imitate him. Dennis could do this so quickly he was making two turns for every one of mine.
"That was fun," I laughed, when we got to the bottom. I commented on his style. "Back in the '80s, I could ski with the best of them," he said. "I'm still getting used to this carving business."

The night went by very quickly. I decided I'd take a night shift whenever one was offered.

# February 2002

## Feb 1

Is it February already? When the heck does winter start? Oh well, I guess we just have to take whatever we can get. Amazingly enough, we've probably only had maybe two days when ski conditions weren't very good. The snowmaking and grooming crew may not look like rocket scientists, but based on the job they've done so far this year, they certainly qualify, maybe not as rocket scientists but certainly as snow scientists. Give these guys honorary PhDs in snowology.

This morning, I was sitting at First Aid Top, engaged in a lengthy, extremely technical discussion on the male reproductive system. Personally, I was hoping the discussion would just naturally move on to the female reproductive system, but it didn't. Eventually, however, we did get around to the prostate gland, and the examination thereof.

I related a story about a doctor I'd gone to for a thorough physical. He'd gotten through most of it. Finally, I heard the dreaded, "Okay, now I'm going to check your prostate." "You should know that I'm subject to passing out during this," I told him. "Okay, then lean to your left," he said.

I asked him what good that was supposed to do. He said, "You're a big guy. You faint, I don't want you falling on me."

This is the same doctor I'd once questioned about my drinking habits. Describing my weekly consumption, I asked him if he thought I drank too much. "The definition of an alcoholic," he told me solemnly, "is someone who drinks more than his doctor. You're fine."

\* \* \*

Kids love Steve Brennan. I do not know why. Personally, I find the guy kind of scary. He stands about 6'3", weighs a good 240, has a shaved head and, depending on his mood, usually has about a 3-day growth of goatee.

Steve also comes complete with a deep scar on the left side of his head, running from the middle of his skull down into his forehead. The way he tells it, when he was a kid, he and his brother used to stand about seven feet apart and whip crab apples at each other. The first one to cry was the loser. One particular day, Steve got the best of his brother, but still had some apples left over. As his brother walked away, Steve got him in the back of the head with a couple more apples. His brother evened the score with a baseball bat, leaving Steve with a permanent reminder of his brother's low tolerance for crab apples.

Kids, for some reason, have no problem asking Steve how he got that dent in his head. His response: "That? That's my rain gutter. Water collects in it and runs down the side of my face. Keeps my nose dry." They buy it, every time.

Today, two little girls walked into First Aid Top, adorable in their expensive little snow-bunny outfits. One said, "We're cold," complete with gestures appropriate to the "princess-in-training" that she is. Steve walked over, got down on her level and growled, "What makes you think I care if you're cold or not." She was taken aback for a moment, but recovered quickly and pointed at the white cross sewn on his pullover.

Steve slapped both his knees and stood up straight. "Oh, rats, you got me," he said. "Now I have to take care of you." The girls giggled. Steve picked one up and walked to the heater, elevating her so she could hold her hands directly in front of the vent. The second little girl came over and planted herself beside them, clearly put out that she wasn't getting any attention. Steve reached down and picked her up too.

A few minutes later, Lee Bates called out that it was my turn to go out and ski. As I walked out the door, Steve was sitting at one of the picnic tables with the girls, playing a silly word association game with them. He was loosing badly.

# Feb 4

All's right with the world – the New England Patriots have won the Super Bowl, the most exciting Super Bowl ever, in the humble opinion of this long-suffering fan.

My friend Brian Murphy, probably a closet Patriots fan, flew in from Dallas in time for the game. He claimed that he was in the area on business and didn't feel like watching the game by himself. Whatever the reason, it was good to see him.

We watched the game at the home of another buddy of mine, Joe Misiewicz, a ski bum who also happens to be a doctor. Joe and his family have an absolutely drop dead beautiful home. As we walked up to the front door, Brian said, "I thought doctors weren't making any money these days." This struck me as funny. Joe's always telling me just that, how difficult it is for a doctor to make a living in today's environment.

As we walked down a few steps to the family room, I noticed a very attractive young woman. She was sitting with her husband, but the old pick-up line, "Don't I know you from someplace?" formed itself on the tip of my tongue, regardless. She beat me to it, however.

We quickly went down the list of all the logical places we might have known each other from. Finally, she hit it. "You don't work at Gunstock, do you?" she asked. "I'm a patroller there," I told her. She laughed. "I work there in marketing," she told me. Her name is Debbie Irwin.

It takes hundreds of people for the mountain to function efficiently, it occurred to me. It's really a small town all to itself. I'm only really familiar with the patrollers, lift attendants and groomers. I hardly even know any of the ski instructors, in spite of the fact that we share a locker room. We come and go on different schedules. Who knows how many back office people I've never laid eyes on.

The folks who make up the ski patrol are a disparate group. We have some lawyers, a doctor or two, and a number of others in medically related careers. And then there are out-and-out ski bums, the guys who work hard labor summer jobs – nothing that might get in the way of skiing. Still, they dream of big houses and hot cars and boats. I've occasionally tried talking to them about saving and investing. Living from paycheck to paycheck, they don't begin to see this as remotely possible. They assume that since I'm already retired, I couldn't possibly understand – or maybe remember – what it's like to have to scramble for money. A few of them will probably live this way all their lives. I doubt they'll feel terribly cheated if they miss out on any of the creature comforts. Food, a roof over their heads (their own or someone else's), money for new skis – that's all they'll ever need.

There are worse ways to go through life. I've worked with people with huge jobs and more money than they could ever spend. They lived to do business, and they were miserable human beings to be around.

# Feb 6

Working the night shift, I had a chance to take care of some regular people stuff today. For starters, I was badly in need of a haircut. My "barber," Beth Silvestri, said she could squeeze me in. Waiting my turn, I listened as Beth attempted conversation with a woman who was obviously hard of hearing. The fact that she was under a hair dryer made conversation all but impossible. Beth kept yakking and the woman kept nodding, but I doubt she had any idea what Beth was saying. Beth has a somewhat older clientele.

I've noticed recently that *my* hearing isn't what it used to be. People who mumble have become especially difficult for me. I realize I find myself trying to read their lips. The long, slow slide is starting. Now that I'm a patroller, I guess it'd be more appropriate to picture it as long, slow snowplow into senility.

I am reminded of a Rottweiler I used to own. As he aged, I could have sworn he was going stone deaf. Still, it seemed he had no problem hearing anything that might be of importance to him. If you so much as whispered anything about food, or taking a walk, he'd be right at your knee. Once, I mentioned to my ex-wife that I had to go to Milwaukee on business. That old dog, zoning in only on the second syllable of the city's name, came shooting out of another room to plant himself expectantly by the door.

So there I was, waiting to have my hair cut. The shop door opened and an elegant-looking woman walked in. I looked up at her, smiled benignly and returned to the copy of People magazine I'd been skimming. After a minute, I took another furtive glance. I didn't want to get caught staring, but there was something about her.

Finally, I had to ask, "Excuse me. Did you grown up in Waltham?" Looking startled, she nodded. "You didn't live on a cul-de-sac across from the Main Street Bridge, did you?" She nodded again, very slowly. I told her my name, to which she responded, "Oh my God, I used to baby sit you when you were three years old."

I haven't seen her since I was four, I kid you not. We talked a bit and discovered that our lives had taken surprisingly similar tracks. She and her husband, having moved all over the country for his career, finally had the opportunity to settle in the Lakes Region of New Hampshire. They'll never leave. When the kids finally get out of college, they'll just slow down the pace a notch.

It's a small world. Or is it? Maybe it's just a case of the older you get and the more you've traveled and experienced, the more you'll come across that's familiar. It's like the deal about time flying as you get older. I read an article that proved why. When you're 48, your frame of reference is just so much wider than when you're four or eight. Time does indeed start to feel as if it's whirling by.

\* \* \*

The night shift was no less eventful than my day. I actually didn't even feel like skiing. I passed on a couple of opportunities to do so, letting others take my circuit. I hope I'm not growing bored with skiing. I certainly better not be. School vacation week for Massachusetts starts in a couple of days.

# Feb 7

The Doug Hamilton rule officially went into effect today. This rule states that no fish or fish by-products can be cooked at First Aid Top.

The weekend crew fancy themselves to be quite the gourmets. Their menu to date has included among other delicacies, a leg of lamb with mint jelly and roast potatoes and a pork loin with an interesting little stuffing. However, this past Sunday Doug whipped up a salmon with wild rice dish. He swears he cleaned the oven when he was done, but come Monday morning, First Aid Top smelled like the Fulton Fish Market. Since then, anything warmed in the oven – pizza, cinnamon buns, whatever – tasted like it was smothered in caviar.

Because of all this, Doug's ancestry has been called into question and/or disparaged. Some of this conversation took place in front of Doug's son Ian, who just shrugged and said, "It was pretty good salmon."

Ian, who looks a bit like Keanu Reeves, is one of the few patrollers here who does the job on a snowboard. It's tough enough pulling a sled wearing skis. I can only imagine what it's like performing this feat on a snowboard. Ian's pretty good on that board. He's very much into the snowboard lifestyle and speaks the language fluently. He can also hear any song and immediately pick up his guitar and play it back for you. Verbatim. He studied the violin as a kid.

Snowboarders and ski patrollers generally don't like each other. They view us as snow cops who just don't get it, hopelessly old and always getting in the way of their fun. We view most of them as roving packs of hooligans ready to attempt any type of jump or flip at whim. Much of what they try to do can – and often does – result in very serious injuries. Every now and then, they run over a skier. Older skiers are leery of snowboarders. In my opinion, it's appropriate.

That said, snowboarders are also the fastest growing segment of the ski industry. Because of this, most mountains cater to them to the greatest extent possible, and Gunstock is no exception. Most of Phelps is set aside as a terrain park, a sort of amusement park for boarders. The park's elements include jumps, half pipes and rails – everything needed for aerial maneuvers in pursuit of permanent paralysis. As part of my regular patrol route, I'll often stop in the terrain park and watch the stunts. I always feel like an interloper.

For snowboarders between the ages of twelve and sixteen, it's not a matter of *if* they'll get hurt, its just a matter of when.

One day Dale Kierstead came across an injured snowboarder sitting in the snow, holding his thigh. When Dale pulled up, the boarder said, "Hey, dude, is my leg supposed to go like this?" He sort of shook his thigh. His upper thigh lifted off the snow, while the rest of his leg stayed perfectly flat against it. Dale told him, "No, it is absolutely *not* supposed to go like that. Please, don't do that again."

The boarder had a broken femur. He should have been screaming and writhing on the snow. According to Dale, he barely made a sound as the leg was stabilized. You gotta wonder what wonder drug that guy was on...

# Feb 8

Friday. Officially, Massachusetts' vacation week starts Monday. Unofficially, it started today. The mountain was much busier than on any normal Friday. Vacation weekdays are pretty much the equivalent of very busy weekend days.

Vacation weeks are huge revenue producers for the mountain. In fact, the profit or loss for an entire season can hang on the proceeds of a single vacation week. Both Steve and Pat have been increasingly on edge as this week's gone along. As members of the management team, they're as accountable for the business angle of things as any of the other managers here who never put on skis.

As the day progressed, the radio sparked with a steady stream of communications as the frequency of accidents increased. Nothing serious, just a manageable, steady stream of incidents. Toward the end of the day, Damon Hodgdon told us rookies, "Everything we've done so far this year has just been a warm-up for next week."

# Feb 11

Today turned out to be the busiest day of the year for the ski patrol. And for me, it will be forever defined by an incident that's convinced me that this is the most fulfilling job I've ever had.

I started out with snowmobile duty, which went surprisingly quickly and easily. Usually the weekend crew writes up a long list of work orders for us, then goes home. Understandably – they're generally flat out on the weekends, at the least the ones I've seen so far. Because everyone knows this is a huge week, I'm guessing that they took care of a lot of stuff themselves.

I got to First Aid Top about 10:00 a.m. Curt Golder was dispatching, non-stop, to patrollers handling incidents all over the mountain. By 11:00, the stream of accidents had picked up, if that was possible. First Aid Top was now staffed by Curt, who was tied to the radio, Karen Colclough, Lee Bates and me.

Curt was on the radio with Derek Whitehead and Pete Henny, both paramedics, who were working on someone with a broken lower leg. The phone rang. I was the closest, so I grabbed it. On the other end was Casey, the attendant at the Summit base. "There's a report of a girl in the woods on Gunsmoke."

"Do you know where?" I asked him. "It sounds like at the Twin Crossover. I think it's bad," he told me. "The guy who reported it was pretty shook up." My stomach dropped.

Thanking Casey, I quickly relayed the information to Curt and started to get up. Curt said, "Hold on. Karen's up next. You'll be second responder." Karen started running around getting into clothes and gear, with Lee at her heels helping her. She was out the door in well under a minute.

In the middle of other calls he was fielding, Curt cued me to get ready and stand by. To Lee he said, "You'll have to stay put so I'm not left up here bare-ass." Or to put it more discretely, there always has to be someone left to respond to another accident. In a worst-case scenario, the dispatcher will go, but that's a real rarity. Lee knows all this. He also knows that Curt's just thinking out loud, trying to stay ahead of things.

In about three minutes, Karen came on the radio. "K-7 to First Aid Top." "Go to Top," Curt replied. "I'm 10-1 at the 10-50, skiers left, Gunsmoke. In the woods." She had a young female with a head injury, status 2, and was requesting a second responder with a backboard sled and trauma pack, and an ambulance. She also asked for as many other patrollers as Curt could provide.

Karen's radio requests usually come in a relaxed monotone. In this case, her communications were stressed, clipped and rapid-fire. In the background we could hear an odd, melodic wailing, almost like a strange birdcall, which became a scream, then retreated back to a wail.

I'd probably have taken the door off its hinges if Lee hadn't opened it for me. I could see in his face that he was aching to be involved in this. I grabbed a sled and jumped into my skis, yelling at people to get out of my way as I ripped down the mountain. I'd never been more serious in my life, and it came across loud and clear. They got well out of the way.

I came to the split between two trails, known as the Twin Crossover, and a cluster of skiers. About twenty feet off the trail, down a steep slope, I saw Karen and another woman, huddled next to a young girl laying supine and thrashing around on the snow. Karen was doing her best to hold the girl down. The girl was still alternating between screaming and that haunting wail we'd heard over the radio.

Shouting to Karen that I was on the scene, I forgot to let Curt know that I'd arrived, but he'd quickly get the idea. Karen yelled back over her shoulder that she really needed the cervical collar. I grabbed it from the sled. Figuring she'd need the trauma pack, I slid that down the slope so it hit Karen in the back. I also got the backboard out and slid it down into the general vicinity. Then I leaped down the hill, landing in snow up to my knees.

The other woman was an off-duty nurse who'd witnessed the accident. Having stopped for a bit of a rest, she was looking back up the hill, watching other skiers, when she noticed this girl traveling at quite a fast clip. As she approached the Crossover, it looked like she suddenly couldn't decide which trail to take. Instead, she went full speed into the woods, impacting a tree with her head, then wrapping her body around a second tree. "It was awful to watch," she told me. I'll bet it was.

Karen kept telling the girl, "Don't move, honey. Don't move." Sometimes this settled her. Other times, she struggled with us. She was tremendously strong for her size. "We've gotta get the collar on her," Karen said. I moved up to the girl's head. Her helmet was still in place.

Just then I looked up to see Lee arriving on the scene, half sliding, half falling down the embankment. I was glad to see him – his seasoned presence was reassuring. He knelt down at a distinctly problematical angle and quickly sized up the situation.

"We gotta get her helmet off," he said. "I'll hold her head. Karen, you get the goggles. Gerry, slide the helmet off." Karen gingerly slid the goggles off the girl's face and up and over the helmet. I gently worked my hands up inside the helmet and stretched it just enough to slowly pop it off. Lee had full responsibility for keeping the girl's head absolutely immobilized. He couldn't move. I could tell he was already uncomfortable.

Karen was just about kneeling on the girl's chest to keep her from flailing around. From this position, she leaned forward awkwardly and started to slide the collar under the back of the girl's head. Seeing it get stuck in the snow, I quickly moved up so I could pull the collar through. Once freed up, it again caught, this time in a huge mass of the girl's long hair. Karen got the hair out of the way as best she could. I pulled the collar around and Karen snapped it in place. It wasn't on perfectly, but it would have to do.

I got the oxygen cylinder, activated it and handed it to Karen, who placed the mask over the girl's nose and mouth. We weren't able to get the strap over her head. Lee said, "If you can get it under my hands, I can hold it in place." He wasn't in a position to make any moves. He was now beyond uncomfortable. I asked if he wanted to switch with me. "Not yet. Keep going," he said.

Karen asked the girl her name, but got no reply. She'd calmed down a bit, but still struggled and cried out occasionally.

Ryan Schruender, another patroller, now appeared at the top of the hill and leaped down into the woods. The nurse had been trying to hold the girl's lower body still. Ryan took over for her. Karen now reached for the backboard. I knew she had her hands too full to do any type of assessment. Someone mentioned that they thought the girl might have broken her leg. I palpated both legs but didn't feel any abnormalities, nor did I get any pain response.

Karen laid the backboard next to the girl. Just as we were all in place to turn her on her side, she started thrashing around again. Lee still held her head, while I leaned a good part of my body weight across her body. Ryan did the same with her legs. She calmed down.

"We gotta get this done real quick," said Karen. On Karen's three count, we turned her and laid her back down on the board. The angle of the slope we were on was working against us. We got the girl situated as best we could. She started to moan. Anticipating that she might try to move, I leaned across her again. She was running out of steam.

Karen started to work the straps around the girl. I told Ryan to help her tighten them down. While he was doing this, I reached under the girl's coat and started to palpate her abdomen. As I pressed on her upper right side, she spoke to us for the first time. "Hurts." "What hurts, honey," Karen asked her. I pressed again. "Hurts," she yelled.

Karen, Lee and Ryan finished getting her secured to the board and tightened down. Lee, finally able to move again, limped around a bit. I looked up to the bystanders. "We could use the help of anyone who'd like to come down here," I called up to them. A boy and a girl slid down the embankment.

"Okay, let's get her out of here," Lee said. I climbed up to where her head was, put a leg on each side of the board and grabbed the handle that was located between my legs. Lee was to my left. Karen and Ryan were at her feet. The boy and girl were to my right. Lee said, "Gerry, on your count, let's start moving her up the hill as smoothly as possible." On three, we all started pushing and pulling, but making very little actual progress. I was thinking we're never going to get this poor little girl out of here.

I planted each of my feet against a different tree and pulled for all I was worth. The others slipped and slid as they pushed and dug and tried to clamber up from below. Finally, Lee grunted, "One more good one should do it." Before I knew it, we were back up on the trail, me ending up in a seated position. Karen scrambled around to put the oxygen cylinder between the girl's legs and make sure the mask was on securely.

Ryan, Lee and the boy lifted the backboard and slid the girl into the toboggan. While they were strapping her in, I popped into my skis and stood between the handles of the sled.

Lee yelled, "Go!" and I started to skate off. With Steve Brennan's lecture on sled-pulling foremost on my mind, I disciplined myself to proceed at a moderate and smooth pace. I radioed that I was transporting the injured party from Gunsmoke and asked that a snowmobile be waiting to tow me in from the flats. I was told that Pat was waiting with the sno mo, and that the ambulance was on site.

Coming out of the woods at the bottom, I saw Pat sitting sidesaddle on his snowmobile. "Hi, Gerry," he said as calm as could be. "What's her name?" I told him we hadn't been able to get it out of her. He leaned over the sled and said, "Hi, honey. What's your name?" "Brenda," she replied. "That's a pretty name," said Pat.

He turned to me to explain, "The oxygen's taking effect." He reached down and adjusted the mask, which had gotten jostled during the ride.

Backing the snowmobile around in front of me, he untied a rope that was coiled around the back of it and threw it over to me. As skiers passed, looking down at Brenda, their expressions turned serious. At the sight of someone wrapped up in a sled with an oxygen mask in place, they assumed the worst.

I wrapped the rope around the handle of the toboggan, then gave Pat the thumbs up. He started to pull us at a slow but steady pace until we reached First Aid Base. I undid the rope and threw it to him, then slid the toboggan down the ramp to the trap door. I took the handles off, then knocked on the door.

Chris Gamache, who I hadn't seen in a while, leaned out and grabbed for all the gusto. Together we pushed and pulled the toboggan inside. I hopped down from the ramp and walked in the door.

The toboggan was already surrounded by Chris, Sharon Hannifan and two EMTs. I joined them. Pat walked in behind me as I gave one of the EMTs a quick update. I told him we weren't happy with the placement of the C collar. "No problem," he said. "We can adjust it now. I asked him if I should cut some of her hair off. He replied, somewhat severely, I thought, "Never cut a woman's hair. What you can do is cut her turtleneck down to the shoulders."

The sled straps had been undone and the canvas wrap was now pulled open. Gingerly, I unzipped Brenda's coat, under the backboard straps. As I was cutting her turtleneck, she opened her eyes, looked up at me and asked, "Who are you?" "I'm Gerry," I told her. "I brought you down in a sled." "Thank you so much," she said, then closed her eyes again.

I sensed that Karen had come in behind us. She pushed her way into the circle. Gently starting to rub Brenda's knee, she asked me, "Have you told them about the response you got from her abdomen?" "Not yet," I replied.

Karen told the EMTs, "When Gerry palpated her upper right quadrant, we got a pain response." Pat went for a stethoscope. Returning, he leaned over, cut Brenda's turtleneck from her waist up to her bra, pulled the material back and started to listen around. Brenda reacted mildly to the cold of the stethoscope. After listening a bit, Pat told one of the EMTs, I have crepitus." Crepitus – the sound of bones grinding against each other, or air crackling internally – is a sign of internal injury.

The door opened behind us. Lee Bates entered with a tall gentleman, Brenda's father. Lee told me later that as he was cleaning up the scene, the man had skied up and asked Lee what was going on. Lee told him there'd been an accident. The guy immediately asked, "Was it a little girl?" Lee responded with his own question. "What was she wearing?" Upon hearing the description, he'd said, "Maybe you'd better follow me."

I leaned down to Brenda. "Look who's here," I said. Her eyes popped open and she exclaimed, "Daddy!" Then her eyes closed again. The poor guy was distraught. "Don't worry, honey," he said. "These people are taking good care of you." He repeated this over and over, clearly trying to reassure himself as well as his daughter.

The EMTs were ready to go. We transferred Brenda to a gurney. As we wheeled her out to the ambulance, I asked her, "Brenda? Are you with us?" She opened her eyes, said yes, then immediately closed them again.

After I helped put Brenda in the ambulance, I felt a need to be with my teammates. I walked back inside. Lee had his arms around Karen, who was crying very quietly into his shoulder. I went over and put my arms around both of them. I said to Lee, "This is the closest I've felt to any teammates in my life." He nodded – I think he might have been a little choked up himself. Eventually he said, "You better get back up top. Curt might still be shorthanded."

I walked out into the sunlight. It suddenly dawned on me that I was as hungry as I'd ever been in my life. I walked to the Summit lift in a daze, and as the chair made its way up the mountain, I was overwhelmed with drowsiness. Adrenaline has a different effect on each of us.

I walked into First Aid Top, trying to act nonchalant, and nodded to the several patrollers now assembled there. They, too, were trying not to appear overanxious. Finally, Craig Laurent broke the ice, asking the question on everyone's minds. "Are you going to tell us or not?" I tried to recall every detail while simultaneously inhaling a ham and Swiss.

* * *

The rest of the day was a blur. Non-stop accidents and incidents. I went out on a couple of minor calls, but everything paled in comparison to the scene with Brenda. I vaguely recall putting a box splint on the leg of a grandmother who I'd found lying down in the parking lot. Karen reached the scene of that accident on a sno mo she'd driven across bare dirt.

Late in the day, all hell broke loose. There were accidents all over the mountain. Curt never changed demeanor. At one point, I was on a chairlift listening to Matt Walsh literally begging for help on the radio. He was on scene with a skier who'd stopped abruptly only to have somebody else ski up his back. While he was waiting for help, Matt's injured skier had gone from Status 3 to Status 2, literally fading in front of Matt's eyes. Curt, with no one left to send, kept telling Matt to stand by. In the meantime, he was scouring his notes to see who might be in proximity with the necessary equipment.

All of a sudden, just like the Lone Ranger, Steve Brennan skidded around the corner on a snowmobile, with a toboggan in tow. Hi Ho, Silver! Matt and Steve got things taken care of quickly. The ambulance, already at the mountain for another call, waited, then did a double carry.

For Curt, 4:00 p.m. came and went. He was still talking, non-stop. As the night crew arrived, Curt threw them right into the mix. At 5:45 p.m. he was finally able to turn responsibility for the mountain over to Tiger Top. At 6:20 p.m. he trudged in the door of First Aid Base to a resounding round of applause. Now that the final member of the day crew was in, we could all go home. Curt had to be the most exhausted member of the shift – and he never left his chair.

# Feb 13

Since First Aid Top has no restrooms, Port-a-Potties are provided right outside the door around the corner. But because they, um, fill up very quickly, we prefer not to use them if at all possible. Which is why all of the guys and several of the women will make a couple of round trips a day down into the woods behind our building.

Early in the year I'd announced, "I know it's not my turn to go out, but I've really gotta go to the bathroom. I need to ski down to the lodge." Lee Bates asked me, "Ya gotta squirt or squat?" "Well, uh, I've gotta squirt," I told him. "Just go down into the woods," he said. "But not directly under the building, whatever you do. Come springtime, we don't need any extraneous aromas floating about in here." The mission was accomplished. Some days, the most hazardous act we're called to perform is the slide down and the hike back up from the woods. On particularly icy days, I wear my helmet.

Today, I was down at my favorite bush. It was easy to find because I take a lot of vitamins. All I had to do was look for the glow in the snow. Glancing around, I noticed that a lot of folks had written, or attempted to write, their K-numbers. "How cute," I thought.

As I started to head back, I saw "K-7" composed perfectly. I was halfway back up the hill when it occurred to me that K-7 is Karen Colclough. How could she have accomplished such a feat, anatomically speaking?

I walked back in and asked, "Okay, Karen, how'd you write your K-number?" Karen looked at me like she didn't have a clue what I was talking about. All of a sudden, Ian Hamilton burst out laughing. "I had a little left over, and a very steady hand," he chortled. "I figured I'd give people something to think about."

Note to skiers: Please don't make yellow snow at our mountain. We have nice, clean restrooms in all our lodges. If we catch you going outside, we'll ask you to leave. There's nothing hypocritical about this. We'd prefer to use the restrooms ourselves. Unfortunately, the job usually just doesn't allow for it.

# Feb 14

The mountain's been busy this week. Since Monday, the number of incidents we've been responding to has dropped dramatically. On the other hand, the courtesy ride business is way up. Starting at noontime, when any of us goes out to ski an advanced trail, we automatically bring a toboggan. Invariably, you'll come across skiers who've had enough.

Today, I loaded three people into the same sled before I was halfway down Gunsmoke. Counting the sled, I was controlling at least 500 pounds. When we reached a flat section of trail, I stopped and told them to get out. Puzzled, the woman in front asked, "Is this the bottom?" "No," I replied, "but if we don't get past this part, we'll never get there." Nestled together very comfortably, they really didn't want to get out. Can't say as I blamed them.

A high school race was in progress on Cannonball. The trail was closed to the public, roped off except for a hitch in the rope that functioned as a control gate, allowing the racers to get under the rope and back to the race start.

About 3:00 p.m., we got a report of an injured racer. Curt Golder was next up and he headed down to Cannonball. After a short while, he radioed in that he had a 15-year-old girl with a possible dislocated shoulder. I was next up, so I went and got a chaise lounge and put it in a regular toboggan. No backboard was needed. I went out the door. Since we were so slow, Lee Bates asked if he could come with me. He was told to go.

We skied rather leisurely down Flintlock, onto Derringer and pulled up at Cannonball where we found a pretty young girl sitting on the snow. Curt had wrapped a sling and swath around her shoulder and chest. The swath was so tight it looked like wallpaper. I thought to myself, "I'll never be able to do a bandage that well." Lee and I prepared the sled.

The girl's coach arrived and knelt down to talk to her. Curt came over and told us, "Her name's Yvette. She's from France. This is the first time she's raced in this country."

As we approached the girl, Lee and I decided we were going to show Yvette just how accommodating American ski patrollers could be. I found myself talking very slowly and very loudly, the way you do to someone who doesn't understand English. "He" – I pointed at Lee, again with great exaggeration – "is going to bring you down." Yvette nodded her head. Very good. I assumed she understood me.

Lee was standing behind me, dusting off his French. I heard him mumbling to himself, "Sleigh ride, sleigh ride – how do you say sleigh ride?" He tried out some words that I recognized as French, but I was pretty sure none of them had anything to do with sleds, sleighs or toboggans.

Curt said, "Okay, guys, let's get her into the sled. Lee, you take her legs. Gerry, you get your hands under her butt. I'll get her around her waist." Why do I always get the heavy part? I slid my hands under her upper thighs and butt. Her racing suit felt very cool and silky. I also couldn't help but notice that 15-year-old ski racers from France have very firm backsides.

On the count of three, we gave the girl a quick lift and settled her into the sled. Yvette leaned back against the chaise lounge. Lee strapped her in, still muttering things like, "la bibliotheque" and "Champs Elysées." I stood up and, yet again, very slowly and loudly told Yvette that we were "going...to...go...now." She looked at me kind of oddly, but nodded again. I got ready to drag the sled, but

Lee announced, "Bug off, rookie. I haven't pulled a sled all week. It's my turn." No sense arguing with the master.

Lee pulls a great sled. It's the snow equivalent of seeing a Mercedes being handled on a smooth road. I skied along a couple of feet behind. Yvette was really enjoying the ride, and I was enjoying Yvette enjoying the ride.

We got to Base, pulled the sled through the trap door and met it inside. Pointing to Yvette's shoulder, I very slowly asked her, "Have...you...ever...hurt...before?" Not looking at me, she answered, "No." Must be shy. I also noted that though she hadn't said much, what English we had heard from her wasn't bad.

Curt arrived and started taking down information on Yvette. Lee told me, "Go see if he's gotten to her home town yet. I've traveled in France extensively." I went and looked over Curt's shoulder.

Her name was not Yvette – it was Annie something or other – and she wasn't from France. Her home town was listed as Hingham, Massachusetts. I turned to relay this information to Lee. Then I turned back to kill Curt, who had moved away from the gurney and was doubled over like someone throwing up.

I leaned in under him. He was laughing so hard he was starting to cry. As he tried to stand up, I jabbed him in the ribs with my finger. He doubled over again. When he finally regained his composure, he stood up and let a big breath of air out with a "whhooo."

"I don't know what made me do that," Curt laughed, "but, damn, it's gotta be one of the best numbers I've ever pulled. You should have seen you guys!" He started to guffaw again, then convulsed and gasped, "After you left, her coach asked me if it was okay for her to be with the two of you."

I'm going to get Curt for this. I don't care if it takes ten years.

# Feb 15

Vacation week's started to wind down. Best I can tell, it's been a successful week for the mountain. Considering that the back yards south of here are green, that's pretty remarkable. People in the industry know that even if the north country is buried in snow, if there's no snow in the big cities, it's going to be a nail biter of a season. People who only ski a few times a year don't think about skiing unless they're shoveling their driveway.

We were all sitting at First Aid Base, getting ready to go out and open up the mountain. Pat McGonagle came out of his office. "We have an update on the girl that was brought down from Gunsmoke on Monday," he said, and went on to tell us that she'd been transferred from Lakes Region Hospital here in town to Dartmouth-Hitchcock with a subdural hematoma – bleeding into the brain – and a lacerated liver. She was in stable condition. Pat didn't know if she'd needed surgery or not.

"You folks did a heck of a job on that one," he told us. "I thought you'd want to know what you'd been dealing with," and walked away. I choked up. Looking over at Karen and Lee, I nodded to them. They nodded back. For as long as I'm able to do this job, I won't forget that little girl.

\* \* \*

The worst thing we dealt with today was just before we headed out. A little girl was walked through the door by her father, holding her left hand in her right one and crying loudly. She'd slammed her thumb in the car door. The thumb had a deep gouge in it, and was already turning purple. Her father was clearly unhappy. He hadn't even gotten to put his skis on.

Pat came out and took a look. He talked soothingly to the little girl while she sat in her father's lap. First he put ice on the thumb, then he broke a tongue depressor in two, positioning a piece on each side of the thumb, and taped it in place. I gave the father directions to the hospital. I'm getting used to dealing with a lot of difference kinds of trauma, but fingers in car doors still give me the chills. As they were walking out, Pat consoled the father. "Maybe you can ski tomorrow," he told him.

We all did a lot of free skiing today. There wasn't much call for us to do anything else.

# Feb 18

Today was the start of New Hampshire's school vacation. Massachusetts and New Hampshire stagger their winter vacation weeks. I'm sure that someone came up with an entirely logical reason for this. Therefore, I don't intend to squander any brain cells in pondering it. Though I can't help imagining the mountains of New England getting together and strong-arming the two states.

As I was driving in to work this morning, I was thinking, "Man, if last week was busy, imagine what this week's going to be like. Every kid in a fifty mile radius will be here." But by midday, the mountain was only a little busier than it would have been on any typical Monday.

I asked Damon Hodgdon what gives. "New Hampshire people get outta town for vacation week, go to Disney World, somewhere warm," he informed me.

"The ones who love the cold head out west to ski. They can ski here whenever they want to."

Damon also predicted it would be a very slow week from the patroller's point of view. "Most of the locals have been on skis from the time they started walking," was his theory. "They don't get hurt like the twice-a-year warrior does."

A lot of us were sitting around at First Aid Top, making small talk. Someone threw out a hypothetical question: "What are you supposed to do if you come across an injured skier who says, 'I'm a lawyer and this mountain's in big trouble?'"

The immediate answer: "Drag him into the woods as far as you can and leave him there." I *think* that person was kidding. Matt Walsh looked up and said, "Hey!" Matt's a lawyer. He went back to whatever he was reading. Somehow, I doubt the article he was scrutinizing was "How to Sue a Mountain in One Easy Lesson."

There's inherent risk in skiing. Skiers are reminded of this from the time they arrive at the mountain. That statement is printed on any number of items they'll come in contact with, in any number of places. You'd think that most people would understand that if they strap a couple of pieces of lumber to their feet and point them downhill, they're pretty much on their own.

I can be a little slow at times catching on to tricky concepts. But I have no problem comprehending that picking up a cobra is an activity that includes inherent risk. If I were to pick up a cobra (for argument's sake, but which I'd never do, considering how terrified of garter snakes I am) and it bit me, it would never occur to me to sue the cobra, or the guy who owned the cobra, or the basket I'd pulled the blasted thing out of.

But people sue ski areas on a regular basis. The law, as it's been explained to me, is that we are responsible for protecting skiers from manmade objects. I write that statement as your humble narrator and not as a legal expert for Gunstock or any other mountain. Manmade objects include (but certainly are not limited to) the parking lot, the stairs to the lodge, the lodge itself, the short order cook, the chair lift, the lift towers, SnowCats, snow guns and the hydrants they get attached to. I guess you could also include other skiers – they're manmade, and I'm sure there are litigants who'd like to include them – but again, for the sake of argument, let's assume that they are excluded.

We sand the parking lot. We sand the stairs to the lodge. We are constantly on the lookout for hazards in the lodge. We know that the short order cook is potentially dangerous, so we keep an eye on him. We have all sorts of qualified people to help you onto the chairlift. We pad any lift tower that stands even close to open terrain. When a SnowCat has to operate on the mountain during the day, it's surrounded by as many patrollers as the President is by Secret Service personnel. And, excluded or not (we take no chances), we knock ourselves out trying to ensure that every skier on the mountain skis responsibly. Still mountains get sued. I'm sure that at any given moment, most ski areas in the country are dealing with on-going litigation.

My personal opinion is that, based on the way we close, mark and protect anything and everything, if some dope doesn't comprehend that there's a hazard up ahead, he deserves to fall in a hole. I'm sure that the dope's lawyer would be very interested in my opinion. I do remind that lawyer, of course, that I'm hardly responsible for formulating the mountain's policy. That's up to Pat McGonagle, the mountain's other managers and the mountain's insurance company.

What I am responsible for is being on the lookout for potential hazards. A large part of a patroller's day is spent pinpointing problems and either fixing them himself or calling someone in to correct the situation. This could be anything from a snow gun that appears to be operating too close to an open area to a tree limb that's potentially threatening a trail. It can be a change in snow conditions, or that the snow ramp at the chair lift off-loading area seems to be a little steep. Subjective judgment calls are a large part of our responsibilities.

As we perform all these tasks, we're not thinking about warding off litigation. We're thinking about the safety and comfort of our guests. The amount of time spent on this kind of work far outweighs the amount of time spent on first aid. I guess you could say that's the point of the exercise. Think of it as preventive medicine for the mountain.

As patroller "numero uno," Pat McGonagle has the ultimate responsibility for mountain safety, and he takes prevention management very seriously. He's constantly spotting things the rest of us just don't see. I find myself wondering if his eyes move independently of each other, in different directions at the same time, like a chameleon. Occasionally aggravated, he'll ask us, "Why aren't you people picking up on this stuff?" Before anyone can come up with an explanation, he'll usually answer his own question with, "I know – you're out here so often that it becomes part of the scenery." But sometimes he doesn't answer himself. Instead, he'll wait for an answer. We do manage to come up with excuses, some of them pretty original. Then we quickly go and fix the problem.

Pat doesn't ski much during the day. When he does, the radio starts burping with his calls, the dispatcher writing as fast as he can, trying to keep up with the laundry list of all Pat's grievances. Pat's list usually includes areas he wants marked off, signs he wants put up or replaced, existing rope lines and fences he wants adjusted or strengthened.

When the workload gets too heavy, we'll occasionally put in a phone call to Sharon Hannifan at First Aid Base. The standard complaint is that Pat's "killing us." She'll then get Pat on the radio and tell him she could really use his help. Sometimes he'll take the bait – even Pat will defer to our "queen bee." On other days, though, he'll come back to her with, "That isn't going to work today." When we hear that, we look at each other and somebody'll ask, "How much time 'til the mountain closes?"

# Feb 20

A little respect here. I'm now a big time TV star.

A couple of weeks ago, a few of us were sitting at First Aid Top, late in the afternoon. The phone rang and Curt Golder picked it up.

"Uh huh. Okay," he said. "Uh huh. Yep, that'll work," and hung up. Everyone was looking at him, curious.

"Anyone want to be in a commercial?" he said, looking right at Craig Laurent and me. Craig and I happen to be very shy – we immediately started to wrestle with each other to keep the other one from getting out the door first. "Children, children," said Curt. "Why don't you both go?"

Craig and I skied down Recoil as fast as we could, obviously both figuring that first impressions would be important. I ski faster than Craig does, but he made the run of his life and we got to the bottom in a dead heat. Waiting for us at the bottom and watching us jostle for position were a couple of guys with a camera and a pretty blonde, of the female persuasion, on skis.

One of the guys told us he used to be a patroller here. These days he produces commercials for local businesses for local cable access. Giving us the once over, he told Craig, "You're just a bit too tall." Too bad. Craig's over 6'4". Then he looked me up and down. I'm just 6'2" "Take off your helmet," he told me. I did. He sized me up like he was some big-shot Hollywood director.

"You'll do," he finally decided. "Do you want to be part of a commercial?" I yawned. "I suppose so," I finally told him.

"Here's the deal," he said. "This commercial's for laser eye surgery. You don't have a speaking part. When the model skis down to you, act like you know her and start talking to her, in a very animated fashion. The X in the snow's your mark. Do not look directly at the camera, and do not look directly at her. Look past her." I nodded. I guessed I could handle all that. He said, "Annnnd, action."

The model kind of wobbled toward me on her skis. It's possible that she'd never been on skis in her life. The cameraman cued me. "Start talking to her." My mind went blank. I couldn't think of a thing to say. However, I recovered quickly.

"I guess the surgery doesn't work. You're blind as a bat," I told her, flashing a big toothpaste commercial smile. She laughed in reply. "You're right. So – are you a guy or a girl?" she asked. I gave a hearty laugh and punched her lightly on the shoulder. The cameraman said, "Cut." They thought it was pretty good. They took a couple more shots from different angles, then we were done.

They started to pack up their gear and head out. I skidded after them on my skis, trying to give them my address so they could send the residual checks. As they got into their car, the producer called, "Thanks again. That was great." They drove off.

I skied over to the chairlift where Craig was waiting for me. "I hope they got my best side," I said, conversationally. "You don't have a best side," Craig informed me.

Curt came on the radio. "K-42, are you guys done down there?" I replied that I would no longer answer to K-42. "From now on I'd like to be referred to as Dirk Dougherty," I announced to all my radio listeners. "Okay, Dirk," replied Curt, "why don't you and your sidekick get your asses back up here. We want to close the mountain. You're holding us up."

Craig and I hopped on a chair and radioed that we were on the last chair for the day, #145. No one will be allowed onto the lift behind us. "Did the camera guy tell you to act like a horse's ass," asked Craig, conversationally, "or does it just come naturally to you?" I told him that jealously doesn't become him.

Well, the commercial started running this morning. It opens with the model staring into a mirror with a somewhat cross-eyed expression. The next scene features an old guy who looks vaguely like me, wearing my patrol coat. He's leering at the girl with a goofy smile. God, I hope this thing only runs once. I hate it. If other commercials are any indication, it will be running every twenty minutes for the next month.

# Feb 22

As part of the patrol job, we have to act as snow police. Some of my teammates hate this aspect of the job. Some love it. Most of us just consider it another aspect of everything we're expected to do. We have the authority to have someone removed from the mountain. If things get really dicey, we have the authority to have someone arrested.

As part of the evening sweep, we push along people who are skiing too slowly. Slow skiers at closing time are referred to as "Bogies." We have no problem with Bogies. They're making it down as best they can. Often we'll help them along by putting our skis into a snowplow V and having them slide in behind us. Their job is to position their skis between our legs and hold onto our waists so we can bring them down. They usually enjoy the ride, and we get them down far faster than they could under their own steam. If that method doesn't work, we call for a toboggan and give them a courtesy ride. We leave it up to them. They may be holding things up, but they've paid for this last run.

"Poachers" – people skiing on a closed trail – are another story. Trails are usually closed for a lack of snow cover, because of hazards that can't be dealt with, or because the trail can't be groomed.

Trails are closed with a bright orange rope laced with a number of flags. A sign that reads "closed" hangs from the rope. In case you only speak Chinese, the sign also carries the universal representation of a skier enclosed in a circle, a circle with a slash through it.

For some reason, we've had a lot of Chinese folks skiing with us this year. I am happy to report that they never ski on closed trails. A lot of the local kids do, though. Based on the number of tracks we find on closed trails, people do manage to get past us. These culprits are usually spotted by a patroller riding a chairlift or standing on an adjacent trail. Their description and location are called to First Aid Top. More often than not, a patroller on a snowmobile is waiting for them at the bottom. Invariably, they're surprised at being caught. They're even more surprised when they're told that what they've been doing is against the law. They're generally a bit more than chagrinned when they lose their lift ticket.

Right now Hot Shot, our most challenging run, is closed off with everything but razor wire. It's still a challenge to keep the poachers off of it.

# Feb 26

Vacations weeks are all over with. The year will start to wind down quickly from here on. Steve and Pat are back to being relaxed, making up for a lot of skiing that they didn't get in earlier in the year. They've even overlooked a catnap or two. Thank God – one of the catnaps they overlooked was mine. While I was dispatching, no less. I was leaning way back in the chair with the sun beating on my face. Don't get me wrong – I didn't sleep through any radio calls. I was more like the parent who's asleep, but still manages to hear every move one of their kids makes. The minute the radio sparked, I'd lean forward, open my eyes and mutter, "Go to top." The guys were calling this my rest mode, like with a computer.

\* \* \*

This morning, Bob, my mailman, asked me, "Did I see you on TV?" "Yes, you did," I answered warily. "Thought so," said Bob. "You looked like you were trying to pick up the blonde chick." Thanks, Bob.

Later in the day, as I was getting off the Quad lift, the lift attendant came out of his booth and asked if I'll stand by. I was hoping he didn't want to talk about TV commercials. He didn't. "I got a report of some kids coming up on the lift," he told me, "who are spitting on people below them. Chair 86."

Chair 23 came around the bull wheel. I kicked out of my skis and we stood and chatted, talking mostly about how soon the season will be over, everyone's favorite topic this week.

As chair 84 came around, I started to move over to the unload. Chair 86 arrived, with three teenage boys on it, two of them on snowboards, the third on skis. I motioned for them to come over to me. The three slid over, looking like the picture of innocence. "Guys, we have a report that you were spitting on people as you were coming up in the chair. Is that true?" I asked, staring hard at them.

The one on skis answered immediately. "It was me. These guys didn't do anything." I had to appreciate his honesty and the fact that he'd fallen on his sword for his friends. I told the others that they were free to go. They backed away just a bit. I turned on the guilty boy.

"That is one of the ugliest things you can do to another person. Would you like it if someone did that to you?" I asked him. He dropped his head and mumbled, "No." "What makes you think it's okay to do here?" I asked. He replied, "I don't know why I did it." "You're through for the day," I informed him. "Give me your pass." He held the pass out from his coat. I cut the wire bale that held it and walked away. The pile of passes at Top is growing.

Three women had been standing off to the side, watching as all this transpired. As I stepped into my skis, one of them said to the others, "They always let them off easy. He should have taken all of their passes." I pretended not to hear her. I did take note of what she was wearing, however. If I came across her later in the day and had any cause to speak with her about something, she was going to wonder why I was so angry.

# Feb 27

Around noontime today, it started to snow as hard as it has all year, the kind of snow I associate with the big mountains of the west, not what we usually see in New England. The snow line started about halfway up the mountain. Base refused to believe it when Top radioed down about it. "It's pouring down here," came the response.

By closing time, we already had five inches. Oh, sure. Now that the year is just about over, it's going to start snowing every day.

Most people wouldn't have thought about skiing today. How could they know that at least half of our mountain was enjoying the best conditions of the year.

We all got out and just plain played in the snow, and squeezed in as many runs as possible. At one point, a couple of us noticed a snowshoe hare nibbling the stalks of plants right next to our building. His coat was starting to go from pure winter white back to its other-seasons mottled brown. At times, he blended right into the bushes. We all just stood around in the falling snow, watching him hop around on his oversized back paws. I don't know if he trusted us or just figured that we couldn't see him. In either case, he wasn't at all bothered by our presence.

Just about sweep time, the snow turned to rain, and our beautiful powder turned to concrete. It was decided that because of this, the mountain would be closed for the evening. Which meant we had to sweep every trail on the mountain. Some of the patrollers were having real problems as we snowplowed down, though for some reason, I didn't. I waited at a checkpoint in the soaking rain for what seemed like forever.

Finally Lee Bates came along, clicked poles at me – and swore. He'd been forced to stop twice to scrape the snow off his skis, he told me. With his knees, he couldn't wait to get off the mountain.

When we walked into Base, Steve Brennan asked Lee how the conditions were. Lee replied, "I survived. I can't comment much beyond that."

# March 2002

## Mar 4

I can't believe how quickly the season is barreling to a close. We were talking today about how long they'll be able to keep the mountain open. Pat McGonagle said, "No problem. These are glacier conditions – warm during the day, cold at night. A little snow in between. We could probably keep the place open till May, if we want to." Amazing, when you consider the lack of natural snow and the warm temperatures.

Truth be told, most ski areas could care less about natural snow. Other than the fact that it constitutes free advertising, it's just not that important to them. By the time decent quantities of snow starts to fall in the east, the ski resorts have already spent tons of money on snow making – depending on the size of the mountain, the cost can run upwards of $1000 per hour. Sometimes those guns run non-stop for weeks at a time. Manmade snow is preferred for many reasons. Primarily, it's more durable for constant grooming, not to mention the fact that it just holds up better in general.

Gunstock has a couple of huge races scheduled for the end of this month and the beginning of April. It would be a huge embarrassment for the mountain if we couldn't make it that far. "I'm telling you, it won't be a problem," Pat keeps telling me.

## Mar 7

After work today, I headed straight for chemistry class. I take the class for 2½ hours, twice a week. I'm not taking it because of any love of chemistry. Not long after my day of working the first aid room and my conversation back then with Pat, I started to give serious consideration to a medical career.

My first choice was to be a physician's assistant. Since I'm realistic about my age, however, I decided I'd have to rule that out – that choice would take several years. I don't want to be starting a second career just when all my friends are starting to retire. My second choice was nursing.

* * *

I called the New Hampshire Technical Institute and asked for the Dean of Admissions. A pleasant fellow named Frank Meyer took my call. I told him I wanted to get into the nursing program starting in September of 2002.

I was sincere, I explained I was older, and I made it clear I was desperate. I was a man on a mission – and I didn't have the luxury of time to play around. He pretty much told me I'd still have to apply like anybody else. He seemed to think I needed to be dissuaded from assuming that I'd just stroll in on my first day of class to a standing ovation. I got the message.

I was told to get hold of my high school and college transcripts and send in an application. "I've got one problem," I told him. "I got a D in chemistry in high school." The Dean went silent for a moment. The prerequisite for admission to the school is a C, at the very least. "Oh. Well, then that's where you start. Remedial high school chemistry," he informed me.

"Doesn't life experience count for anything?" I asked. "Nope," he answered, "but a B in chemistry would." He then helped me get hooked up with the Laconia adult ed coordinator and into the required course. It had started three weeks previously. My "real" nursing courses wouldn't start until the fall, but for me, this chem course was as real as it gets, a huge step for me.

An exam was scheduled a couple of days after I started. I was told I could put it off a week, but I figured I wouldn't know any more the following week than I did already, so I took it. I got a 74. There was certainly room for improvement, but at least I was in the game.

Night instructors seem to get it that night students are a serious bunch, with a distinctly different brand of motivation than their day students. Night students are mostly people who've chosen a path, often a bit later in life, and are pursuing it under less than ideal circumstances, simultaneously holding day jobs and in many cases raising a family. Upon occasion, night instructors will cut their night students a little slack.

Everyone in the class appeared to be there for the same reason as me – they'd gotten serious and decided they wanted to go into one form of medicine or another. Either they'd never taken chemistry, or like me, didn't get the point of it the first time around. After a number of quizzes and labs, my grade is now hovering at a B+. I am determined to get an A.

# Mar 12

I got to the gym at the ungodly hour of 5:00 a.m. this morning. Dean, a regular, kept me company. He's always here when I arrive. Today, he already had a good sweat going for him. He greeted me with, "I've really had a good workout today." Finally, I just had to ask, "So what is it? Are you an insomniac or what? What the hell time do you get here?" He ducked his head and laughed, then replied, "I really don't need much sleep. Plus I've got a new puppy who wakes up about

3:45. I don't want to wake my wife up, so I get up and put him out. Then he and I sit in the La-Z-Boy and watch the Weather Channel. I'm usually here about 4:30 a.m."

Dean owns a large crane he uses to take down trees. I bet he can't sneak catnaps. There was one on the agenda for me today, that was for sure. I left the gym at 6:05, a good ten minutes before my usual gym buddies arrived.

I was on the mountain at 7:00, first one in. Big deal. I live less than three miles from here. Most of my teammates have a much longer commute, some more than an hour. On snowy days, those trips can turn into two hours or worse. With a tip of the hat to empathy, I assure them that I never leave home in the morning without listening to the traffic copter – gotta know what kind of road conditions you're dealing with. On bad days, they don't appear to appreciate my sense of humor. Today was a bad day, icy and slushy. The conditions on the mountain weren't much better. We weren't expecting much of a crowd.

The march towards the end of the season continues. When I first started, we'd have to rush to get sweep completed before darkness fell. Now we've got plenty of daylight left when we're done. I'm starting to wish we could close tomorrow. We're doing far too much sitting around. Even skiing doesn't hold the same allure it did a week or two ago.

I'm told by the veterans that everybody contends with these sentiments, this time of year. Every time we pick up a few more inches of snow, I find myself saying, "Damn. That's another few days we'll be open." Pat's right. This place isn't going to close till May.

# Mar 13

Before work today, I went for my second in a series of Hepatitis B shots. They don't hurt. It just means going to the occupational health center and waiting in line. It's strongly recommended that people in the health services receive these vaccinations. In my opinion, it ought to be mandatory. Hep B and Hep C are becoming not so silent epidemics.

As I was wearing all my work clothes, I asked the nurse if she wanted to just shoot me in the butt. She said, "No, it has to be in your upper arm." Struggling out of several layers of clothing, I found my modesty around medical people had hit an all-time low.

I used to be a totally modest guy. I have a cousin in the medical field who used to bring up what most of the rest of us considered the most inappropriate subjects at the dinner table. I've just started to notice that I'm doing that myself now.

We sometimes have to get injured skiers into various states of undress so we can see exactly what we might be dealing with and address it. Our main concern is for their dignity – we do everything we can so they won't be embarrassed. I find, however, that seriously injured people could care less if you stripped them naked. All they care about is for the pain to go away.

## Mar 15

We have some serious gourmets on the full-time shift. Curt Golder is one. Damon Hodgdon's the other. Damon's worked as a cook in a restaurant – he's not a chef, but he's worked with one. Clearly he took very good notes. Damon assured me once that he could go through the garbage and come up with enough stuff to turn out an entirely passable meal. So I got up and looked in the garbage. I'm not sure what he'd make out of peanut shells and Milky Way wrappers, but I think I'll believe him anyway.

Curt's the cook at home every night, which sits just fine with his wife, his dog and Curt. Today he brought in a Mexican chicken dish with spicy rice, enough for everybody. Oh, man, it was good. So good I was hoping the lift would break down, so I could have the portions of the patrollers who were on their way up. I didn't think the drool on my chin was all that noticeable, or maybe it was the way I was sitting on the edge of the couch ready to spring, but Curt finally patted his thigh and said, "Here, boy. Bring your dish." I got seconds, and I wasn't shy about it, either.

Next week he says he's going to make us something Chinese, and maybe, if we're lucky, something Italian. Yum yum. I remember when I used to feel this way about girls.

## Mar 20

We had six inches of snow today. On top of three inches yesterday. The place is going to be open until the 4th of July. In addition, the groomers have started moving large amounts of snow from low traffic areas to high traffic ones. It's almost as if they'd planned this way back in the beginning. Well, shucks – I bet they did plan it.

The door to First Aid Top swung open and a guy walked in, threw his arms wide and announced, "Steve Barnes is back!" Everyone jumped up to welcome him. I vaguely recognized him from the recertification weekend, back in November. I hadn't seen him since. In November he was sporting a large brace on his leg.

By most people's estimation, Steve Barnes is the prettiest skier on the patrol. Not in looks but in style – he's one of those skiers people just like to stand and watch. Two years ago, Steve was doing some back-country skiing with friends when somebody accidentally cut him off and he hit a tree, at full speed. His lower thigh and knee took most of the impact. His leg's now full of hardware, and he's been engaged in extensive therapy for a year. Today was his second day out. He admitted it was coming back slowly.

At the age of 19, Steve was the youngest patrol director in the country. He'd applied for work at an area in northern New Jersey – Steve's a Jersey boy. As it turned out, the area had let its entire staff go the previous day. They asked Steve if he thought he could supervise people. Like I said, he's a Jersey guy. What do you think he'd say, "No?" He said, "Sure." Then they asked him if he knew any other patrollers he could hire. So Steve put together a team and became the youngest patrol director in the country.

At the end of each winter season, Steve would head down to Argentina or Chile and patrol in the Andes for the summer. I asked him if he enjoyed that. He said, "Oh yeah. That was a blast. I also learned pretty good Spanish." Since a lot of the guests were the "beautiful people" from Monte Carlo and the like, I can only imagine what else he learned.

He now has a successful business. His wife and daughters are waiting for him outside. On the 1 to 10 scale, they're right up there. What is it with some guys?

# Mar 27

Yesterday, we had four inches of – you guessed it – snow. Today we had early summer. Temperatures in the flatlands reached 70 degrees. This meant we had great skiing until about noontime, then it slopped up, big time. The potential for knee injuries went way up by late afternoon. I decided early in the day that my knees weren't going to be among those put at risk. I resolved I'd only ski when told to, and if told to, I didn't expect to be too enthusiastic about it.

What I did do with enthusiasm, however, was drag a couple of couches outside and help feed the radio and antenna out through the window. We could now all sit out and work on our tans, with plenty of skiers getting off the Summit lift for entertainment. Some of them had truly interesting dismounting styles. Occasionally, one or another of us ran over to pick someone up and brush him or her – okay, her – off. About once an hour, somebody forgot to get off altogether and started to go around the bull wheel. A gate automatically shuts down the lift in this event, which sends Erin scurrying out of her lift top booth to help the person down. We usually all run over to help Erin. We like Erin a lot.

We had such a luxurious day that no one wanted to leave. Plans began to ripen that revolved around getting a keg of beer and a barbecue grill sent to First Aid Top. We decided that we had sufficient accommodations for us to have a sleep over. All of this fell through when Pat McGonagle stepped off the lift at 4:12 p.m. and started chasing people around with a ski pole to get sweep started. Oh well. It was a good plan.

# April 2002

## Apr 3

Today I made the first mention to anybody that I'm keeping a diary. It came up while a cribbage game was in progress. Somebody swore and I said, "Watch it. I'm keeping a diary. And I should tell you – I'm quoting actual conversation." The players looked up, and the player who'd sworn said, "That's nice." They went back to their game.

Later on I was riding up on the chairlift with another patroller. I told this individual that I'd been keeping a diary and that I might explore the book avenue. This patroller's first reaction was, "I hope you won't hurt anyone."

"That would absolutely be my last intent," I said. The patroller considered this, then said, "Please don't use my name in anything. Especially if you write about my love life."

That's a fair request. I won't use the patroller's name. However, I do have to say that this patroller's love life is perfectly awful.

## Apr 5

Today, Friday, was my last day of work for the year. The mountain will close at the end of the day on Sunday. After wishing for this day to come for the past several weeks, I found myself sad and nostalgic now that it had actually arrived. Lee Bates tells me my reaction is typical. We had a very slow day, with only one incident involving a broken ski pole, but no bones.

Riding up the chair lift in mid-afternoon, I started to contemplate the past several months. I thought back to the first day I walked into training. I've come a long way, with barely time to realize it. There have been tremendous highs, and with them, some very low points. All in all, I am so glad that I basically fell into this. I hope I'll be able to do it for a long time to come.

At the end of the day, we turned in equipment. Emptying out my jacket, I found a buck thirty-seven in one pocket and another fifty-two cents in another. I also pulled out a pair of non-latex gloves and some seriously creased skier responsibility cards – I gave out maybe two of those all season.

As I exited the building, I stopped and took a long look up the mountain. The sun was still shining off the top. I tried not to be too melodramatic, but this I wanted to remember.

# Post Season

# April 2002

## Apr 7

At 5:00 p.m., I arrived back at the mountain, which 45 minutes ago closed for the year. The parking lot was empty. Today's patrollers were just coming down from their final sweep. I was here for the year-end patrol party.

Walking towards First Aid Base, I found "Chef" Damon busy scraping down the grill. Two toboggans were parked on the ramp, loaded with ice and beer. I chuckled to myself – I contributed a bunch of that beer, with all my various little slip-ups. Pat McGonagle, snapped a picture. "I'm going to send this to the manufacturer," he said. "I'll bet they never thought of this use for their sleds."

There was at least a ton of food. I pigged out, to use the technical term. The only concern I have about my weight these days is getting it back up. When I started classes in September, I weighed 225. I bottomed out at 206 and am now closing in on 212. This job is so much more demanding than I'd ever realized. At 206, I had a washboard stomach. The downside: none of my clothes fit. Ah, the annoying tradeoffs of life.

The party grew progressively festive and loud. The tunes were cranked way up. Ian and Doug Hamilton played some beautiful numbers on guitar and fiddle. Pat McGonagle eventually raised his hands to get everyone's attention. "We've got some awards to give out." The place quieted down a notch.

"First off," said Pat, "is Rookie of the Year. That goes to Gerry Doughterty."

Stunned, I just sat there. "Get up there," Curt Golder stage-whispered as he elbowed me to my feet. Dazed, I made my way up to Pat, who shook my hand heartily. "You got 20 out of 25 votes," he told me.

I went back to my seat to a nice round of applause. Karen Colclough gave me a hug. "You were the natural selection," she said. "But I screwed up so much stuff," I said, still mystified. "You always tried so hard," she said.

Driving home, I reflected on the whole experience. This was a great year. I am so glad I signed up, and made it through both the rigors of the course and the realities of the season.

The enormity of it all was just beginning to sink in, now that the season had officially come to an end. I've learned so much. I've discovered I have a natural ability for some aspects of the job. I've finally gotten on top of other aspects that took me so long to learn. Tomorrow I'd get to sleep in.

# Apr 8

I walked into the gym at 6:25 a.m., a much more normal, human-type time to be there. The regular crew was in attendance: Uncle Al, Regular Al, Tommy, Jose, George, Joe, Lee and Cindy. I hadn't seen any of them in a while. Tommy looked up. "Nice of you to stop by," he said. "Mountain's closed, huh?" Gilford's a company town.

Closed indeed. Now I can get back to my normal routine. A nice leisurely workout first thing in the morning, followed by breakfast, followed by a nap. Errands, followed by a nap. A couple of hours of wrestling with chemistry, followed by – you guessed it – a nap. I can also catch up with the two or three episodes of M.A.S.H. I don't have committed to memory. The reruns are on all day. Lately, I find myself wondering if my decades-long infatuation with M.A.S.H. wasn't a symptom of some inherent predilection for medicine.

Most of the group at the gym are bikers. They make a point of getting to all the major events every year, the highlight of which is the trip to Daytona in February. About once a week they assemble their "Over The Hill Gang" and go off on a long ride. They'll stop, have a nice lunch and knock back a few lemonades, whatever.

A while back, they suggested it was time I bought a bike and joined them. I told them this was a great idea, except for one little wrinkle: I'm afraid of motorcycles. Nobody made fun of me for this admission. Uncle Al put it best, "If you know that about yourself, then you probably shouldn't ride. Motorcycles ain't toys."

Bike or not, I get invited to their parties. I usually go. One of the first I attended was a cookout. The whole gang was there. I recognized National Hockey League coach Pat Burns among the crowd, who I'm more used to seeing in a suit on TV In his biker attire, he looked big and tough. At one point during the evening, a couple of Hell's Angels stopped by for a cheeseburger and some small talk. They also looked big and tough. I'd never seen them in a suit.

I found myself thinking, "Now this is an interesting group of people. Here I am in my penny loafers, dry-cleaned Levis and Polo shirt. I look like a total dork." But my friends could have cared less. All that concerned them was that everybody was having a good time and getting enough to eat. As a group, they're much less judgmental than most folks.

# May 2002

## May 8

My father came up the cellar stairs and into my living room this morning. "When are you going to do something about the grouse?" he asked me. "She just attacked me in the driveway."

I'll explain the grouse later. First let me explain my father, who came into my living room on crutches. He's been on crutches since he was in his early twenties. In July of 1945, his left leg had to be amputated at mid thigh.

My father worked in the engine room of the *USS Underhill*, a destroyer escort that was cruising with a convoy of ships off the Philippines in the South Pacific. About midday of July 24th, they got into a lively situation, to say the least: a periscope was spotted and it was decided that the *Underhill* would ram it.

But before they ever got the chance to pull off this maneuver, the ship was ripped in two by a horrific explosion. She'd been rammed at the artillery magazine by a Japanese two-man kamikaze sub. Moments before the blast, a friend of my father's had come down from above deck yelling, "Frank, go topside. It's a wild show." The last thing my father remembers is heading up those stairs. Later that day, his friend turned up dead. My father didn't do all that much better.

Every July since the end of World War II, my father has made a pilgrimage to the Naval Academy in Annapolis, Maryland, for a reunion of the *Underhill* survivors. As time passes, the list of attendees has started to dwindle. In 1995, my father asked me if I'd go with him. Up till then, my mother had usually accompanied him, but she'd died earlier that year, on January 31st. I assured him I wouldn't miss it for the world.

At the reunion, I got to talk with guys I hadn't seen since I was a kid. This was the first time that some of their stories really meant something to me.

One of my father's best friends on the ship, John Macky, was a genuine character. My father has always kept in touch with him. These days, John, or Macky, as he's called, drives the Zamboni at the Erie, Pennsylvania, ice arena.

Macky recounted his recollections of that day. "One minute I was sitting at a big gun," he told me. "The next minute, I was about two hundred yards away, in the water, with all of my clothes blown off. The ship was already going down."

The fellow who was chief medic told me, "I was worried about people who were going to live. Your father just looked like a big pile of dirty rags hanging from the ceiling." At some point, Norm McCarty, another friend of my dad's, looked up and said, "Hey, Chief, that pile of rags just blinked its eyes."

All of this wouldn't be much from a historical standpoint, except for one thing: the cruiser *Indianapolis* – the ship that, on one of the most secret missions of World War II, delivered the atomic bomb.

The *Indianapolis* dropped off her deadly cargo at an island near Guam, then turned around and started to steam back to San Francisco. If someone had told her skipper that the *Underhill* had been blown up 85 miles away, a whole bunch of people might have been much better off today – most of her crew never made another port. The same "mother sub" that was responsible for sinking my dad's ship came across the *Indianapolis* a few days later.

In the middle of the night, a couple of torpedoes blew *Indianapolis* out of existence. The only survivors went into the water. Since she didn't officially exist, no one came looking for them. The survivors floated in the South Pacific for several days before they were found by accident. A PBY search plane spotted a huge oil slick and went in to take a closer look.

My father was just regaining consciousness in a hospital in the Philippines when they started bringing the *Indianapolis* guys in. He told me that a lot of them were dehydrated and delirious, and their skin was hanging off of them, from being submerged in salt water for so long. Some had seen their best buddies blown to bits. Others had watched as sharks came and nibbled at the limbs of people floating right next to them. If you want to read about what people are capable of surviving, there are now a number of books out about this particular affair.

In any case, my father's been a weekly visitor ever since my mother died. Among other things, he's my gardener. I won't say he's got a green thumb, exactly, but the place is always tidy and colorful. He never lets his handicap get in his way. Occasionally, I come home to find him on the roof repairing shingles. I have no doubt that if he were a few years younger, I'd have him skiing right beside me.

My mother once told me about their early days together. She met my father on a blind date. His ship was docked in Boston. She was very pretty, and admittedly very naïve, and she'd been on one too many dates with rough and rowdy sailors. One look at my dad, however, and she knew this guy was different. She told me that between the time he shook her hand and cleared his throat to speak, she'd decided she was going to marry him.

She didn't hear from him for a while. Then one night, my grandfather went into her bedroom carrying a copy of the Boston Evening Globe. He put the paper in her hands, then grabbed her for all he was worth. The headline read, "*Underhill Sunk, With 212 Aboard.*" They sat together for a long time.

Eventually my mother found out that my father had survived, though with life altering injuries. She didn't hear much else.

Several months later, my mother went into Boston with a friend, a couple of girls out on the town. They went to an area known back then as Scollay Square, one of Boston's more colorful "combat zones." (You won't find Scollay Square on the map any more – urban renewal took what was left of it in the 1960s. Today it's the site of Boston's City Hall.) Crawling with hookers, burlesque houses and sailors looking for a good time, this was certainly not the kind of place my mother normally frequented.

The two girls ducked into a little shop for a cup of tea, where, for a dime, you could have a "professional" fortuneteller read your tea leaves. They were there to have fun. The gypsy fortuneteller was exotic. My mother went for it.

After a few minutes pondering my mother's teacup, the gypsy looked up at my mother quizzically. "Who's this one-legged man? You will see him again," she told her quietly.

For the rest of her days, my mother would have nothing to do with anything that smacked of fortunetelling. She wouldn't even read her horoscope.

I digress.

And while I'm digressing, one final footnote: when my mother was diagnosed with terminal cancer, it was agreed that she should die in her own house. A bed was set up in the dining room, and a visiting nurse came twice a week. For the most part, my father took care of her.

As always, he refused to let his handicap get in the way of what was the most selfless time of a selfless life. With the help of my cousin Karen, who's a nurse, he cared for his wife to her last minute. He tied a little bell to her hospital bed for her to ring whenever she needed something. The bell was a little replica of the Liberty Bell. They'd bought it for me when we visited Independence Hall, back when I was seven. She rang that bell early and often. He never missed a third ring.

My father's the most private and unemotional man I've ever known. He may be displeased when he reads a couple of the previous pages. He doesn't like to have his life hung out for the world to see. The last time my mother rang that bell was about thirty seconds before she took her last breath. My father was there. For maybe the first time in my life, I understood true love, something I hope that I am capable of.

\* \* \*

Now about that grouse. The grouse in question's a nasty bird that's taken up residence in my yard. Nasty? This bird's possessed. She's lived there for about two years now.

This grouse looks like an unholy cross between a pheasant and a hawk, weighs about ten pounds, has beady eyes, a crown of feathers on her head and earth-toned camouflage coloring. When she stands still in the woods, she's almost impossible to spot. If only she'd stay in the woods.

She first announced her presence one day as I was taking grocery bags out of the car. I looked around. There she was, astride a stone wall, glaring at me. Ever since then, she's become increasingly bold. Given the opportunity, she'll attack the windshield of the car, as I back out of the driveway. She regularly chases me into the house.

One day I was in the woods, stacking wood, when I heard the familiar rustling of my nemesis working her way towards me. But this time I was prepared. I had a sawed-off hockey stick with me.

This infernal bird hopped up onto the pile of wood I was working on and hissed in my face. I grabbed the hockey stick, locked eyes and jabbed her in the chest. The bird didn't flinch. Instead, she stuck her chest out as if to say, "That doesn't bother me one bit, pipsqueak. Try it again, though, and I'll kick your ass." I immediately went into the house and called the Audubon Society.

The woman on the other end of the line was sympathetic. "This is all very typical grouse behavior you're describing," she assured me. "Happily, we have no record of a grouse ever actually harming a human being. Why don't you just see if the two of you can co-exist?"

I told her I was only too happy to co-exist. Unfortunately, the grouse was giving no indication that she was willing to sit down and negotiate. "Unfortunately you are living in her territory," the Audubon lady explained patiently. I told her I'd been living in what I considered my territory since well before the grouse first came along. She asked that I try not to hurt it. Hey, what about me?

Initially the grouse only had eyes for me – she'd rush past anybody else to chase me around. My father found this greatly amusing. "Maybe she was a house pet," he offered. "Maybe you should feed her." "Sure, Dad," I answered him. "This is a vicious, wild animal. Trust me, the last thing I'm going to do is feed her."

Recently the grouse has started charging my father. Picture a man on crutches, trying to run from a ten-pound bird. At least he no longer views the situation as amusing.

This creature had better mend her foolish ways. I have a lot of friends who are hunters. She wouldn't look half bad under glass, with a presentation of cranberry sauce.

# May 17

I don't like to brag. Well, okay, that's a lie. I got an A in chemistry. I took the pre-nursing boards and scored in the top fifth percentile.

The school continues to request more information. I could have sworn I'd applied to N.H.T.I., not Dartmouth. I'll have to go back and find out where I sent all that admissions stuff.

I've had time to seriously ruminate about how I spent my winter.

I used to view Gunstock as the little neighborhood mountain. I skied there fairly often, but I'd get bored and go off to find bigger adventures. But I always found my way back.

Now that I've worked there, I've developed a profound respect for our little neighborhood mountain, and all the people it takes to make it operate. I have an intimate knowledge of the place. Suddenly, it seems much bigger to me than it used to. And I'm not writing that to suck up to anybody.

Common knowledge says that familiarity breeds contempt. But not always. Sometimes, like in a good marriage, familiarity can breed more love. I love Gunstock. I hope that I'm still allowed to hang around there if this thing ever gets published.

As a skier, you shouldn't have to think about what goes into making your experience enjoyable. You should pull into the parking lot, look up at the slopes and say, "Ah. This is going to be a great day. I'm going to take some incredible runs." You should expect nothing less – you're spending a lot of money for the privilege. It takes hundreds of people to bring your expectations to fruition. The ones I know take their responsibility for the success of your visit very seriously. Over the course of the past months, I've become well acquainted with emergency providers. Whether their primary careers are as doctors or ditch diggers, they have one thing in common: when they come across a person in distress, they want to make things better.

Folks who decide to pursue this vocation are people just like you, with the necessary training and an affinity for the people they serve. When they arrive at a ski wreck, they don't know what they are going to find. Sometimes they laugh. Sometimes they want to cry, or throw up. They rarely do either of the latter in front of you – that's for later. I hope I've been able to get across to you some of what goes into these jobs.

I want to go to nursing school very badly. I'm still waiting to hear. I see "ER Nurse" in my future. I hope that happens.

If it does, maybe I should keep a diary.

# The Making of a Physician Assistant

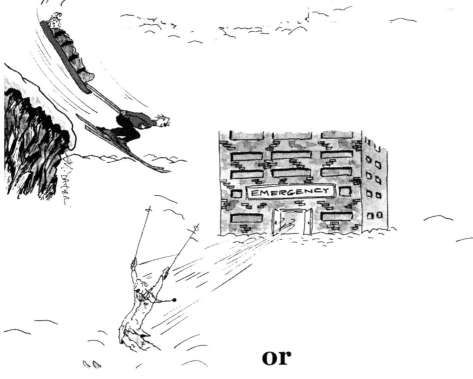

or
how I turned a
**pipe dream** into **reality**
in just a couple of years!

# Another Introduction?

You want to know why you're reading a second introduction, right? Okay. Fair question.

What you're getting here is basically two books in one, so the way I see it, that entitles you to a second introduction – all for one money. What a deal!

The first part, the ski patroller story, was supposed to be the be-all and end-all. I'd never intended anything beyond that. But, as it turns out, that was just step one towards what has become the career of a lifetime – at least for the remainder of *my* lifetime.

Getting through the training that brought me to the first day of the career of my lifetime, however, was the equivalent of skiing a big-time bump run. Just like any hairy run, there was fun and plenty of it along the way. But there were also some super scary moments, the kind where you find yourself wondering how on earth you ever thought you knew what you were doing – you know the kind.

When I first started skiing, if you took one of those falls that left equipment all over the mountain, it was called a "yard sale" – today you'd call it a "digger." A couple of times along the way, I took the emotional equivalent of your choice of those, but there's no question it was all worth it – plus it's given me the opportunity to expand the number of pages in this book and, holy cow, raise the price!

Part I was written while in the throes of learning, a diarist's reflections on a day's runs at the end of that same day. Part II, which chronicles my passage through the mogul-strewn steeps that took me from patroller to physician assistant, was written after the fact, degree safely in hand, in contemplative retrospect.

If you enjoy reading this half as much as I enjoyed writing it, then I believe you will have gotten your money's worth. I hope you'll find yourself wanting to read it a couple of times!

Gerry Dougherty
Gilford, N.H.
August 16, 2006

# Nursing School

I got into nursing school at New Hampshire Technical Institute. The day that I got the "Congratulations. It is with great pleasure that we offer you acceptance..." letter, was one of the high points of the spring. I would start the nursing program in September, 2002. I decided, since I was already in somewhat of an academic mode, what with my great success in remedial high school chemistry, that I might as well go to school all summer. I already learned from my hiatus from the workplace that I really wasn't going to be missing much if I spent my summer in a classroom.

I popped in to see my old friend Frank Meyer, the Dean of Admissions who'd been so helpful in getting me started down this road back in January. Like most of the staff at the school, he was very pleasant and helpful. He didn't really remember our earlier conversation but he could tell I needed to be led by the hand. He got me where I needed to be to register for Anatomy, Physiology and Intro to Psychology. I had taken Psychology during my first time round in college and had gotten a C. NHTI was willing to give me credit for that and a pass on having to take it again. I decided to pretend like I'd never been to college (some professors from my first four years would most likely agree with that assessment) and start fresh.

I tackled the academics with a vengeance. I had something to prove to myself. It didn't hurt that I really liked both the material and the professors. I spent most of my waking hours away from the classrooms with a book in my hands. It started to pay off. The A's started coming. The day after my second anatomy exam, Craig Meservey, the professor, walked by me and said, "Your grade on the exam was ridiculous." Uh-oh, I thought. "Not good?" I got up the courage to ask. He said, "Just the opposite. Including the extra credit question, you got a 107. Ridiculous." He smiled and walked away. Maybe I should just become a full-time student until it was time to collect social security.

The summer went by quickly. I got to know many of my fellow students, about 80% of whom were getting ready for the nursing program; the rest were headed for dental hygiene. A minority of them were just out of high school or undergraduate programs. Most, like me, were attempting a second career far different from their first one. We couldn't wait for the real deal to get started.

Nursing school started at 9:00 a.m. on the day after Labor Day. I found my way into a hot amphitheater jammed with people headed in all directions. I slowly worked my way up the steep stairs to an aisle seat about half-way to the top. I knew from recent experience that the seat you claim would be yours for the semester. I liked this one. After a bit, everyone more or less settled into place. I gave the room the quick once-over. There looked to be about 120 or so students, 11 or 12 of whom were guys. Ages ranged from about 19 to me. Virtually everyone carried backpacks – except for me. I had my leather Saatchi briefcase, a vestige of my days in the toy wars.

Once everyone got themselves more or less situated, we were called to order. A large woman with glasses and mostly strawberry blonde hair had taken the podium, introducing herself as Barbara Dunn. I figured that she was the 'major domo' around this place. (She wasn't). I had a feeling she might be someone who it would be worth getting to know. (She was).

Barbara started off by congratulating us for picking such a noble profession – and telling us that we were about to begin the toughest two years that any of us would ever experience. I sat there thinking, "Bring it on!" I was soon to learn that she wasn't kidding. Most of the day was administrative: where to go, when to go and what would be expected of us when we got there. We also discovered that they weren't going to waste any time before throwing us into the hospital environment. Clinical rotations would start the following week.

The following day we were back to meet with the nurse who would be our advisor while doing our hospital rotations, and to get our assignments. My advisor was a soft spoken, easy-to-smile fellow named Patrick Hornig, a nurse practitioner who had worked in an office environment until he'd gotten fed up with being pushed to see patients at a rate that didn't allow him to spend time with any of them. He was now going to show all of us how to be a nurse. Good luck to him.

After a quick week of classroom time that involved learning about drugs and procedures and which end of the bedpan to put under a patient, it was time for my first day in a hospital. As I drove to Concord Hospital at 6 a.m., I was sick with nervousness. I found myself wondering what the treatment for diarrhea was; I was pretty sure that I was going to have a bad case of it. I walked into the main lobby wearing my white running shoes with my white pants and my half-length white student coat. I considered announcing my arrival by saying, "quack, quack." The fact that I didn't see Patrick or any of my fellow students didn't make me feel any better. Before I knew it I had two matching half moons of sweat coming through the underarms of my coat.

Eventually my classmates began to straggle in, most admitting aloud that they felt pretty much like I did. Patrick came around the corner in his full-length white coat, carrying a big mug of coffee. He took a big gulp. The site of all of us huddled together seemed to amuse to him. He said, "Lets go get oriented." We formed up in a cluster and followed close on his heels – quack, quack – to a room where he went over what he expected of us, then reviewed hospital codes and regulations. We finished by signing a couple of forms that had to do with patient confidentiality.

Clearly, if you ever got caught talking about a patient in the halls or in the elevator, you'd be thrown out of school and possibly sent to prison.

Patrick said, "Let's head up to the floor. Everybody relax. This is going to be fun." I couldn't hear him; the ringing in my ears from nerves was drowning him out. We took the elevator up to six north, my home one day a week for the next couple of months.

As a student, you qualify as slave labor, and you exist at the absolute bottom of the pecking order. The janitor and nurses aids are supreme beings compared to you. Nurses are generals – nursing students are privates. Medical residents, nurse practitioners, physician assistants and doctors inhabit another universe altogether. Everyone within the medical community has a clear understanding of this and treats you accordingly. Some medical providers look at you as if you were an annoying fly; others act as if you simply don't exist. As a nursing student you try not to get in the way and you speak only when spoken to. When someone extends some basic courtesy or actually speaks to you, you find yourself feeling like you should lick his hand, like a dog who has been beaten too often.

We had already been given information on the patient for whom we would be responsible. Patrick matched us up with the nurse we would be shadowing. My nurse had 4 or 5 patients that she had to deal with, so introductions were on the run. She seemed kind of neutral about my presence. I took the shadowing part quite seriously. I followed her into the kitchen, into each patient's room, into the medication room. I was just about to follow her into the bathroom when she turned around and said, "Look. Why don't you go in with your patient and see if there is anything you can do."

As a student, the morning routine typically consists of introducing yourself to your patients, then checking their vital signs, i.e. pulse, blood pressure, respiration, temperature, oxygen saturation, weight, and extent of any pain. You then do rudimentary physicals, change their bedclothes, help them with toileting, bathe them, and administer medications as called for. Medications are given under the close observation of your clinical advisor. Patrick was extremely cautious with us. At this stage of the game I could barely pronounce the names of half of the drugs, let alone know what they were used for. Patrick spent a lot of time saying, "Look it up," and I spent a lot of time trying to find the drug manual. Typically, what a nurse could do in a minute took me half an hour to accomplish.

On this first morning, however, I didn't get to do any of these things. I knew already that my patient was a middle-aged woman in the end stage of pancreatic cancer. For the purposes of this narrative, we'll call her Jane. I walked in to the room to find her sitting in bed rocking back and forth with hers arms folded across her stomach. I quickly introduced myself and asked her if there was something that I could do for her. She said, "I'm in so much pain." I went and told the nurse who said, "She's had a lot of morphine already but I'll give her some more." The morphine was injected into her IV line which was already in place. It seemed to have minimal effect, but at least Jane started to rock a little slower. About ten minutes later, Jane coded. She stopped breathing and then started again very sporadically. An alarm in her room was pressed. People started arriving on the run with equipment, breathing tubes and needles. As serious as all of this was, I also found it exciting. I tried to stay well out of the way, but I was taking it all in. After a little while Jane started to come around and her color improved. Once she was fully conscious again she immediately stated how much pain she was in. It was decided that more morphine was too risky. I asked her if she wanted me to rub her back. She said, "Please."

I sat on her bed (a definite no-no which was overlooked in this case) and rubbed her back for about forty minutes, until my arms got too tired to carry on. When I stopped she thanked me softly and sincerely. I could tell that I had provided her some measure of relief. I had a tremendous sense of fulfillment that my minimal involvement had provided someone comfort and was appreciated. I helped transfer Jane to the intensive care unit. She held my hand on the way there in the elevator. As we left her I thought, "She's not going to live long enough for me to see her again."

The rest of the day was uneventful. As I left the hospital on this first day, my head was spinning with all the new experiences I'd survived. I couldn't wait to call Christy, a young lady I'd been seeing recently, and tell her all about it. However, as I started relating the goings on of the day, I choked up and couldn't talk for a while. Christy sobbed softly on the other end of the phone.

* * *

The second week started. To the many hours of lecture we now added simulation lab, where we were taught, and attempted ourselves, the procedures that are part of the daily nursing routine. Simulation was taught to us by a nurse named Simone; it quickly became known as 'Sim with Sim.' The room was set up like a hospital emergency room, with a number of bays separated by draw curtains. Lying stoically on each bed was an anatomically-correct crash dummy. These patients suffered in silence while we clumsily practiced inserting feeding tubes and catheters, and performed other procedures that would have caused live patients to scream bloody murder. We also learned to give injections by drawing water up into syringes and giving foam-filled pillows a shot. The pillows were very brave.

You might want to skip this paragraph if you're faint of heart or easily offended. One day Sim was discussing the proper method for relieving someone who has an impacted bowel, a situation when someone has become so constipated that someone, usually a nurse, has to apply a gloved finger to remove some of the bowel's content. I raised my hand and I asked, "Is this something we'll be doing on a regular basis?" Sim wanted to know why I asked. I told her that her answer might influence if I continued on this career path. She laughed – sort of – and said that it was probably done more often in nursing homes than in the hospital environment. I decided to stay for another day.

* * *

Before I knew it another hospital day rolled around. I experienced the same nervousness and sweating, and I could now give directions to every bathroom in the hospital. I stayed up late the night before a clinical to do the tremendous amount of preparation involved. I had to prepare all sorts of care plans. At the time, I thought a lot of them were archaic. People don't stay in hospitals for long these days; a lot of what I was preparing had to do with long-term care. However, what I thought didn't matter much. This was all part of a process, which I discovered as the year went along, was a way for the faculty to control you, giving them countless opportunities to point out how inept you were and emphasize why you would never make it as a nurse.

Patrick, however, continued to be encouraging, helpful and kind. Occasionally aggravated, he would say to whomever was the cause of his irritation, "I know that you don't know what you're doing, but at least try to *look* like you know what you're doing." Usually though, he was in good humor. He could be very funny and a fair amount of laughter was tolerated. He also tolerated my habit of spouting off with any wise-ass comment that came to mind, some of which was straight impudence, pure and simple, I now know, coming as it did from a lowly student. I guess he understood that I was older, with life experiences and a prior career. Either that or he just found me funny. I noticed as the year went on that he was looked down on by other faculty for being too easy on us.

I gave my first injection, to an elderly gentleman with diabetes. Before lunch he needed his insulin shot. Usually when a nurse is about to give a shot they tell the patient, "Little prick coming." I always felt like they were referring to me when they said that. I decided to try a different tact. I thought that, maybe, if I snuck up on him he wouldn't even notice. While I was talking to him about the Patriots' most recent game, I suddenly jabbed the needle into the back of his arm. He said, "Owww! What the *hell* are you doing?" He started swinging his arm around with the needle still in it. Patrick, standing next to me, started shouting to me to grab it and inject. I did. The patient had really liked me up to that point. We left the room. Patrick shook his head and walked away.

Exams started coming one after another. I was doing pretty well on the academic end of things. However, I did badly on one exam and was asked to go and meet with my academic advisor. She asked what had happened and I told her that I guessed I had just studied the wrong stuff and that was I really pissed at myself. What I wanted to say was, "Those were some of the stupidest questions I've ever seen. A number of them had nothing to do with reality," but since I was quickly learning to keep my mouth shut in this business, I said nothing. She asked what had drawn me at this time in my life to the field of medicine. I told her that I found fulfillment in dealing with people in distress and that I liked the idea of diagnosis. She replied, "You're not going to do any of that in this end of the business."

For a while I had been aware of a small voice asking myself every so often, "Do you really want to be a nurse?" I knew that I loved the interaction with the patients and I could tell that most of them liked me. Patients often told me, "You are going to be a good nurse." I knew this had more to do with personality and interaction; I was barely proficient at most procedures. While I had no problem with putting my hands on people, I did not care for the bedpans, bed-making and bathing. This is far from all that a nurse does, but they are certainly a part of things. I refused to let the voice gain ground. I had decided to be a nurse and, dammit, I was going to be one.

I had a patient in clinical that really got to me, a gentleman who had lung cancer that had metastasized to his brain. He had lost the ability to hear, speak, or even blink his eyelids, which were sewn shut. I found that tough to take. He occasionally grunted and struggled to get out of bed. I spent the day taking care of his basic needs and also putting my hands on him a lot so that hopefully he would sense that he was not alone. At one point Patrick said, "His mouth and tongue are all dried out from the way he is breathing. You could make him feel better by applying some moisturizing gel." I put a glob of gel onto a gloved finger and rubbed it all around in his mouth. It was like putting your finger into the mouth of a baby. Later his son came into the room and we talked about how difficult this was for him and the family. His son said, "A couple of months ago he was vibrant and enjoying his daily walks through the fall woods. Look at him now." I put my arm on his shoulder. Later we all met for our end-of-clinical day meeting, where we each related what we had done that day, what procedures we had accomplished and what we had learned. I went last. As I started to talk about my patient, I got a lump in my throat and my eyes misted over. I had to stop talking. Patrick and my mates were very understanding. To this day, it amazed me how that patient affected me the way that he did.

* * *

The semester was coming to a close and I realized that I was starting to learn a fair amount. My grades were good and I was on my way to an academic Phi Beta Kappa rating. I wasn't loving clinical days, but I was getting through them. At the end of the semester Patrick gave me my review. He basically told me I was doing okay. I had some areas I needed to work on, but he told me I was where I should be at this stage of the game. I went home for a nice long Christmas break and some serious ski patrolling.

It was great to get back to Gunstock and catch up with everyone. They were all encouraging about my new career and wanted to hear all about it. Mostly I just wanted to ski and relax. I did a lot of both. Also, since I was becoming more comfortable with the job of patrolling, I handled a fair amount of wrecks that were now actually feeling routine. As the month of vacation started to run out of days, I started to get that nervous, queasy feeling again. Clinical days were just around the corner – and would now be increased to two days a week.

* * *

It was turning out to be one of those brutally cold winters that we get in New Hampshire every couple of years. If you live in Virginia you'd consider any winter in New Hampshire to be brutal, but this was one of those relentless ones, the kind even natives notice. Some mornings my car would just start to warm up at the end of my thirty-five-mile drive to the campus.

One morning I stopped in to see Barbara Dunn. Since that first day when she'd addressed the assembled masses, I'd gotten to know her a little bit. Although I never had any direct contact with her other than attending her lectures, her door was always open. I found her easy to talk to. My attempt at this second career, similar to her own history, seemed to factor into the way she always made time for me. I felt I could talk to her openly and honestly. After exchanging the usual pleasantries about the holidays, she asked me how I was doing. I told her that I liked the program but was still not comfortable during clinical days. She said, "Look, you can do this. Everyone is nervous during clinical. Keep your head down and do what we ask of you. Besides, your next clinical instructor is a great teacher. You'll have a great experience."

Prior to starting the semester I had asked around a little bit about my next clinical instructor. While Barbara's assessment of her was not unique, it was definitely a minority opinion. Mostly what I got were rolled eyes or a sincere "good luck."

Lectures started and seemed to be endless, far more complicated and involved than first semester, but at the same time they seemed more interesting, delving into the whys and wherefores of various disease processes as they did.. Occasionally I even understood what they were talking about. I always assumed the nurses who lectured us were completely knowledgeable authorities on their subjects; when someone knows a lot more about something than you do, I think that's the prudent viewpoint. However, one day we had a lecture on cancer from a nurse that most of us didn't have much to do with. It became evident pretty quickly that she didn't have a good grasp of her subject matter. When students started asking her questions she started looking for the exit signs. I think I knew more about cancer than she did only because I own stock in a company that makes cancer drugs and have always made a point of reading the annual report. I started thinking that she probably got by on most things by flipping her hair and wiggling her gluteus maximi. That was probably the only time I felt that way during the entire year.

Ah yes. Time for hospital rotations and the nerves routine had arrived again. This time I would be at Catholic Medical Center in Manchester. I got to the lobby a half hour early and awaited the arrival of a new group of fellow students and our esteemed advisor. I've decided not to use her name, not for legal reasons or anything, but because her name makes me think of her face and her face ...well, just think of Nurse Ratched in *One Flew Over The Cuckoos Nest*. You remember, the look she'd give Jack Nicholson with her eyelids at half mast and the "I've just bitten into something disgustingly sour" grimace. I got to know that look well.

Our Nurse Ratched bustled into the lobby that first day demanding to know why several students weren't there yet. It was still ten minutes early. No warm greeting, no smiling. I thought immediately, no joking around on this rotation. My days with Patrick immediately became just a fond memory. We finally headed up to the floor for a day that consisted, pretty much, of rules and regulations. As we were leaving she said she expected precise, buttoned-up care plans but that she didn't want us staying up all night doing them. Well, that's reasonable, I thought.

That was the last time I got to think about reasonableness. The next seven weeks were pure hell. Don't get me wrong – she was tough on everybody. Initially I thought, "Well, maybe she's just the Bobby Knight of nursing." As time went on it occurred to me that I was becoming her pet project. She answered most of my questions with a sneer, if at all. By the end I decided that she probably moon-lighted as a prison guard.

I didn't think she was much of a teacher, but she was a great catcher and I gave her plenty to catch. The more I felt pressured, the more pressure I put on myself to get it right. That made things worse. I came to feel like I was moving in slow motion. I started making stupid mistakes, like leaving bed rails down and not placing call buttons where a patient could easily reach them, which only got me more trouble and more pressure. I had never experienced anything like this in my life and that included a lot of years in some very tough business environments.

One night Christy and I were having a long talk. She said, "I'd have no problem if you left nursing." I looked at her like she had two heads. She said, "I've never seen you like this. You aren't funny. You aren't confident. Your whole personality has changed." She said, "I hate these people for what they're doing to you, and I don't like what you're doing to yourself." I refused to listen to her. I did the psychological version of the kid who puts his hands over his ears and goes "la la la la." I was going to be a nurse, dammit!

* * *

It got worse. A patient who had just had her gallbladder removed was hooked up to a piece of equipment that allowed her to have a measured amount of morphine every hour, at the press of a button every time she had pain. If she got to 5 milligrams or whatever in an hour, it stopped dispensing any more.

My advisor came along and asked why the patient still had access to the pain meds. I figured that if you just had surgery you'd be in pain so I said what seemed to me to be the obvious, "Because she's in pain." She said, "No, she's not." I asked her, "How do you know?" She said, "I just told you. She's not in pain" We went a few rounds like this, then finally she said, "I asked the patient if she was in pain. She told me she's not." She walked away. At the end of the day the advisor asked me to join her in a conference room. She asked me, "Are you one of those people who questions everything?" I replied, "I'm one of those people who learns by asking a lot of questions." She said, "I've never been challenged by a student in that manner, *and* you did it in front of other nurses. I'm outraged." I honestly hadn't thought that I'd been challenging anyone. I just didn't get a concept and continued to question. Now I was angry. I wanted to say, "Screw you," or perhaps give her a poke in her smug face. Instead I groveled and apologized for the misunderstanding. I didn't feel very good about myself on the ride home.

I was determined to complete this Bataan Death March. Dammit, I was going to be a nurse, etc., etc. Somehow I managed not to let the patients know how badly I was feeling. Most of them seemed to enjoy my attention and a little humor that they probably weren't used to getting in this environment. As this rotation came to a close I felt like I was just hanging on by my fingernails.

The day came for our end-of-rotation reviews. I was talking with a fellow student named Mikky Toth, who'd come in for some rough treatment from our advisor but felt like he would get by. I told him, "Mik, I'm pretty sure she's going to throw me out." He said, "Nah, I'll bet she lets you slide by."

I walked into her office. She said, "I want you to leave this program. You aren't good at this and you're going to hurt someone." I replied, "I would feel horrible if I hurt someone, but I know that it's a possibility that a student will make mistakes." I added, "You can throw me out but I'm not leaving voluntarily." She shuffled some papers and kept shaking her head. She said, "I'm going to pass you. Barely." She added, "I'm going to try and get you back for another rotation later in the year" The thought of that didn't thrill me but I said, "fair enough," and walked out of her office. I felt about as low as I could get.

What I didn't quite realize yet is that once they've decided that they want you out of a program like this, sooner or later you are going to be leaving. They admit well over a hundred students every year and I'm pretty sure their intention is to get rid of about forty to fifty percent of them.

Craig Laurent from ski patrol was going out with a really nice woman who was a nurse. One night over a couple of drinks I started to tell her about what I was going through. With most people I was pretty close-mouthed. She told me, "Nurses eat their young." I said, "They eat their old, too." She told me that when she was in school she would go home every night and cry, and that she thought she'd never make it. I knew the feeling.

For the moment, I reveled in the breath of fresh air, my good fortune for having escaped. My next rotation would be in a psychiatric hospital. That was fitting – I had just missed ending up in one as a patient. Most students dread the psych rotation, but I was looking forward to it. I had toyed with the idea of becoming a psychologist during my first go-round in college; I'd been interested in the subject ever since. My new advisor was strict but kindly, treating us with a certain amount of respect. The care plans here were different and involved a certain amount of creative writing. If I may humbly say so, I'm not bad at that sort of thing, so I did somewhat better in that department. I was on a floor with younger patients who were considered relatively non-violent. Still, the first day among the general population is a little disconcerting. We didn't do any medical treating here. We did a lot of observing and talking to patients. On the first day I was talking to a fellow student, Melissa Gravilla. A patient with wide eyes came up to me and without saying anything made a complete circle around me as if making an assessment. The impression I got was that, if I'd tires, he would have kicked them. He then moved on.

Prior to this rotation, I had never knowingly been around anyone who was bipolar or manic. I sat and talked to a young guy who was. His eyes were very large and his face gleamed. He waved his arms and used his hands a lot when he talked, rather like my Italian aunts. His speech pattern was rhythmic. He told me that he had many deep and incredible thoughts. I asked him if he could tell me about them. He said, "No. They are not for you to know." I think he felt that I probably wasn't up to it. Dealing with someone in that condition is very hard. People who are bipolar appear to function as if they are on a natural high. You are asking them to take drugs that will bring them down. Many don't want to come down.

It also occurred to me that many of the psychotic episodes that these folks were dealing with were due to drug use. I hadn't realized that LSD had made a big comeback on the street. I wondered if an occasional flashback was being mistaken for a psychotic episode. I asked one of the psychiatrists about this and he said, "That's an interesting postulation." Psychiatrists talk differently than other doctors. This doctor, soft spoken and introspective, was very interesting to be around. He looked like what you'd want a psychiatrist to look like. He even stroked his chin while thinking, like they do on TV.

The best part of the rotation, other than excellent food in the hospital cafeteria, was group meetings. That took up a large part of our day, discussing each patient, their progress (or lack thereof), and their treatment regimen. I liked the team feel of our group meetings and the fascinating conversations that took place therein. Each team had a psychiatrist, psychologist, social worker, nurse and a couple of students. Our team also had a medical resident who was becoming a psychiatrist. I asked him if he had started out to be a shrink. He said, "Nah, I was going to be a surgeon. Then I did my psych rotation. The hours were good, you didn't have to do call, and you could make some decent money. What's not to like?"

One day in the team meeting the psychiatrist was stroking his chin and postulating about a certain patient. He had several very interesting but involved theories about what might be going on. The psychologist looked at him for a minute, then suggested, "Maybe the guy's just nuts." That was the hardest I laughed all year.

One day I walked onto the floor and could feel a tension I hadn't felt before. Several patients were crying, some were agitated and others who were usually easy to control were being difficult. Suddenly a general melee broke out. Security people came running from all directions. I'm quite confident in my ability to handle myself physically but I did what we had been instructed to do in these situations: I made sure the other students were with me and got out of the area to a secure location. When we were allowed back into the area, all was peaceful and calm had returned. I remember describing it at the time as being like a thunderstorm in the summer. Once it passes the sun comes out and the air is fresh.

I liked this environment and started to think that I might like to get into this end of things if I got through this program. The money wasn't bad and I knew that they were always looking for nurses.

* * *

Sadly this rotation, the most enjoyable so far, came to an end. Now I would be headed back to Catholic Medical Center for another round on a med/surg floor. That voice in the back of my mind had surfaced again and was starting to seriously question if I wanted to be a nurse. I knew that I liked the medical field. I was starting to look enviously at doctors and was kicking myself for not having gone that route the first time around. Of course there was a minor impediment at the time. Something about grades. But I was occasionally being honest with myself, giving recognition to the fact that there were many aspects of nursing that I simply didn't like. Then reality would set in. I'd say to myself, "You're too old to go to medical school so get through another year of this program, get a job in nursing and then learn to like it. Besides, what the hell else are you going to do?"

My grades were still decent, but they'd begun to slide a little bit. I decided that for the last month of the school year, I'd kick it up a notch and finish with a flourish. That included my hospital days, which again were twice a week. I was starting to not trust most of the faculty but my new clinical advisor seemed easy going enough and had a certain amount of class about her. On the first day she asked each of us to write one page about ourselves and be honest and open about our feelings about what we were doing. No one would see them but her, she told us. I made two mistakes. The first was in actually doing this project – none of my classmates turned it in. The second was in being completely candid about my mixed feelings. I imagine those sentiments were never far away whenever she dealt with me.

In any case things started to go smoothly. I was feeling better and more confidant, though my hands occasionally shook when doing certain procedures. I thought to myself, "Well, you're not the best one around here but you're starting to get it." At this time we were beginning to handle multiple patients, which involved multiple preparation. On the day before clinical we'd be given a sheet with enough information to prepare for each patient. I thought it odd on one of these days when I only got a sheet on one patient, but I certainly walked in the next day prepared and confident. When my advisor asked why I was only dealing with one patient, I told her that's all I've been given. She said, "Uh-un, you've got another one." That completely threw me. I would have to learn about the patient on the run. I wondered later if perhaps I'd been set up. Was I starting to do well enough that they might have to pass me and used this to throw me out of whack? I decided that I was just being paranoid, but you can get that way in this type of environment.

This same day, one of my classmates stumbled out of a room as white as a ghost. I walked over to her and asked if she was all right. She was on the verge of tears and said, "I just gave the wrong meds to the two people in the room. I switched them." Another student came over and we calmed her down a bit. We kept telling her it was an honest mistake, but we weren't really sure what the penalty would be for this. She made the long trudge to find our advisor and told her what she'd done. They went and reviewed what medications had been given and it was decided that, fortunately, it wasn't that big a deal. These things do happen pretty regularly both to students and nurses. An incident report is filled out after it's been determined that there's been no ill affect on the patient. I remember thinking at the time, though, that if I'd done this I would have been immediately marched out of the hospital under police escort.

I never really got back on my game on this day and I made some mistakes. A patient came back from having a procedure in surgery with an empty IV still hooked up. I didn't notice it and got written up. Again, with the same patient, we were checking vital signs every ten minutes to make sure she was coming around after her procedure. Because I'm tall I raised her bed up so I could listen to her lungs and take her pulse. At one point I left the bed in this raised position, putting the patient at increased risk for injury if she were to fall out. My second write-up of the day. At the end of the day my advisor asked me to go for a cup of coffee. I don't drink it but it seemed like the thing to do. She asked, "How do you think you're doing?" I replied that although I continued to make some dumb mistakes, I felt that I was starting to get it. She said, "I want you to go home over the weekend and think hard about whether you really want to do this." She said, "I have never seen anyone as hard on himself as you are." She asked that I meet with her on Monday morning.

I knew that the end was near. I felt a little bit of relief. I decided that I would let her tell me what the deal was going to be, and that I wouldn't fight it if it was sayonara for the kid.

* * *

It *was* sayonara for the kid. She said that she had thought about me all weekend. I didn't believe that for a second, but it didn't really matter. She thought it was best if I took a hike. So I signed the dismissal forms and took a hike. I drove home and had a couple of martinis. I then laid on the couch, stared at the ceiling and said over and over, "Now what the hell am I going to do?" I asked Christy if she still wanted to be involved with such a failure. I viewed this as being fired. I'd never been fired before. She said she was relieved that I was out, even though she knew that I was disappointed. I decided to allow myself twenty-four hours of feeling sorry for myself. I did a darned good job of it, too.

# Plan B

Two days later I had a plan. I would become a physicians assistant. Lisa Sutherland, who I worked with on ski patrol, had just finished school and was a PA. She was always telling me that I should apply to her school and do the same thing. She kept saying, "You're no nurse. What the hell do you want to do that for?" She went on to tell me that as a PA you did a lot of things that a doctor did, that you definitely practiced medicine. I'd filed all this away and never given it much thought, because the prerequisite courses were similar to med school. I would have to take tons of chemistry and related courses. No way.

However. Now I was on a mission. It was May, 2003. The next class that I could enter would be January of 2004. If I really worked at it, I might just be able to pull this off. Between now and then I would have to take two courses of straight chemistry, biochemistry, microbiology and the bane of many  an existence, organic chemistry. Oh, yes, and some advanced algebra also. I had to get at least a B in all of them to be accepted.

I went back to NHTI to see how many of these courses I could take there. They offered all of them but organic chemistry, it turned out. One problem though: their science courses were pretty much held in reserve for their nursing and dental hygiene students. I would have to get the permission of the head of nursing to get into the classes. I trudged off to a building I didn't like being in. The wounds were way too fresh.

I met with the department head. For some reason she always put me in mind of Cruella Deville, maybe because she so often made me feel like one of those Dalmatian puppies she was always trying to do in. She asked me what I was going to do. I wasn't telling many people and I sure as hell wasn't going to tell her; I was still quite paranoid and in fear of having my plan derailed. I told her I was just going to take some classes and see where it led me. She said, "Why don't you go to work as a nurse's aid and then reapply to this program." I felt like telling her to stick a bedpan up her wazoo, but being the diplomatic guy I am, agreed that reapplying was a consideration. She gave me the approval that I needed.

I would take all of the chemistry and algebra over the summer. I would take microbiology in the fall. Now I had to do something about organic chemistry. I called Plymouth State University, about forty miles north of where I lived. They had openings in the fall in organic. I was in business. I submitted my application at Massachusetts College of Pharmacy and Health Sciences for their PA program, to start in 2004.

My summer days and nights were spent in a classroom. I was a man on a mission and once again had the blinders on, so I didn't know if I was coming or going, if it was day or night. I took all of the chemistry under the same professor. Perry Seagraves and I got to know each other well. He introduced himself as a geek. He said he loved pocket protectors, that he'd use a slide rule if he could find one. He looked like a geek. His hair went off in twenty different directions and he squinted through oversized glasses he constantly pushed up the bridge of his nose. He was a fanatical Red Sox fan, so a lengthy discussion of the previous night's game was required before any class could begin. He included questions about the Red Sox on most exams.

At one point during the summer he told me, "I spend more time with you than my wife. I just don't like you as much." His wife came in to teach us during chemistry labs. Another time he told me that he thought I probably had more chemistry classes than he had taken and "I'm the professor, for God sake."

Perry was also a bit of a mad scientist. He was always saying, "Watch this." He'd mix up some powders, then add a solvent or something. The end result, quite often, was a pretty colored flash, sometimes a small explosion and usually the room would fill with smoke. He would immediately follow all this with, "Don't tell my wife that I did that." He made chemistry as fun as it can be, which isn't very. His philosophy was that chemistry is what it is. It doesn't matter if you're studying it at Harvard or NHTI – it's all about how it's taught. He taught it well. Towards the end of the summer I asked him why he didn't teach organic chemistry. He said, "I don't like it." I asked, "Didn't you have to take it?" He replied, "Yeah, but it was no big deal. All of the pre-med students sat in the front row scared to death that they would fail it and not get into med school. All of us chem majors sat in the back and threw paper airplanes at each other."

\* \* \*

Before I go much further, I feel that I should address a couple of things about my nursing school experience. First, in hindsight, I can now look back and realize that those folks did me a favor. I'm not thrilled about having been demeaned and belittled by some of those people but they were right – I didn't belong in nursing. With enough experience I wouldn't have been a bad nurse, but neither would I have ever been a happy nurse. Nursing wasn't where I belonged.

Secondly, for anyone who ever deals with a nurse, I have some advice – repeat after me: nurses run hospitals. They may not be the executives of the place, but hospitals do not – and cannot – function without them. You will have a much better hospital experience if you are polite to the nursing staff you encounter and try not to demand too much of their time. They are very busy, categorically overworked and definitely under-appreciated. It might appear that nurses are well paid, but that's not really the case, considering all that they're responsible for. Also many of them are truly physically beaten up by the demands of the job. I love nurses. There are just a couple of nursing instructors that I can't say I was too thrilled with.

Considering the workload I had taken on, my grades were pretty good. All A's and a B in advanced algebra. When I consider just how much I hate math, that might have been my greatest accomplishment through this period.

It was now time to tackle microbiology and organic chemistry. Organic chemistry is one of those subjects that you either get the concept or you don't. A friend of mine who was retired from a very successful career in business told me that he had started out to be a doctor. Organic chemistry finished off that dream. According to him, the professor told him one day, "I'm going to give you a C under one condition." My friend asked what that was. The professor said, "That you don't come back."

Right after Labor Day I took my first trek up to Plymouth. The school sits on a beautiful little campus nestled in the foothills of the White Mountains. My class was held in a attractive amphitheater in Plymouth's brand-new science building. My professor, Dr. Davis, was a wonderful gentleman who I believe has since retired. He was also a doctor of organic chemistry, so he bordered on being a god in my eyes. The only problem I had with him was that he talked on a level that most of us couldn't attain. It came so naturally to him that it probably never occurred to him that we students didn't have a clue. The class was at eight in the morning, three days a week, with a three-hour lab once a week, after which I would rush the fifty miles down to NHTI to take microbiology under Pat Yokell, a professor I'd already experienced in other classes. I liked her a lot. I consider her to be simply one of the best teachers I have ever had the pleasure of learning from. A stickler about timeliness and classroom etiquette, she could occasionally do some pretty well-deserved yelling, so some students weren't too keen on her. Personally, I loved her.

Even though I was running around a lot, this schedule was a breeze compared to the summer, plus we were getting into my favorite time of year, fall and early winter. I was struggling in organic, so I stopped in for a chat with Dr. Davis. He told me that he didn't think I was doing that badly and besides, he said, "You show up every day and you ask good questions. I'm pretty sure you'll get a decent grade." He also told me that he greatly admired what I was attempting to do at this stage of my life. I felt better.

I did miss one day of organic, the day I went to Mass College for my interview. I hadn't worn a suit coat and tie for a while and it felt uncomfortable. I walked into the building on what I hoped would soon be my campus. A whole bunch of young people were sitting in the lobby looking all washed and dressed in their best threads. Varying degrees of nervousness were on display. I wasn't nervous at all. I viewed this as a job interview and I had always done pretty well with those. Plus I was a man on a mission. Also, I had a secret weapon: my mother had died in 1995, and I was starting to believe that she'd been pulling some strings for me recently. I was starting to see too many coincidences that were going in my favor.

The time came for my interview and I was escorted into a room where two faculty members awaited. Both PAs, it turned out that the guy would be leaving in December. The woman was Gale Furey. She was blonde and attractive but definitely not what you might call perky – cocky was more like it. They asked about my background and my schooling. After several more questions, Gale asked, "So why do you want to be a PA?" I said, "I know that a paycheck goes with the job, but I'd do it for nothing. Dealing with people who are in physical or emotional distress is the most fulfilling thing I've ever done." (My current employer should not read too much into that no-pay part.) They both started scribbling at the same time. During my years of selling I'd honed the skill of reading things upside down that people were writing at their desks. In this case, unfortunately, I couldn't see what was being written, but my gut told me it was good. Gale said, "If we accept you into this program, it will be predicated on your getting good grades in the courses you are currently taking and you must shadow a PA for fifty hours." I had known about that part but had pushed it to the back burner. Now that time was running out, that would have to become a priority.

I was then ushered into another room, along with several other candidates. The two faculty members who awaited us here explained that they'd give us a scenario involving an ethical dilemma which we would need to work out as a group. I knew they wanted to see how we interacted with each other and how forceful our individual personalities were. They were also on the lookout for jerks. I quickly reminded myself not to monopolize the conversation. However my years in business kind of kicked in. I had been in several jobs where I was usually the one in the room doing most of the talking. I also had often been the one doing the consensus building between people from different departments in companies. So my own evaluation of the ethical dilemma simulation is that I was a little bit of a loudmouth. Months later, one of the folks in that room confided that, although I was now one of her favorites, she hated me that day. Still I walked out of the building feeling I'd nailed it. I called Christy and told her I was pretty sure I was going to get in. I could swear I could hear her jumping up and down through the phone.

Now I had to find a PA in my area who I could talk into letting me stare over his or her shoulder for fifty hours. None of the PAs I knew personally worked locally. Even though my schedule wasn't horrible, I was going to have to work this in, and I figured I should make it as easy as possible on myself. I happened to run into a woman that I'd been with in nursing school. I got around to asking if she knew any PAs. She said, "My primary care provider is a PA. He's great. Call Mirno Pasquali."

I went home and immediately called Mirno's office. I got through to him immediately, which threw me a little. I explained what my deal was and he said, "Yeah. We can get that done. Come in next week."

\* \* \*

Mirno Pasquali is one cool guy. He has a great head of salt and pepper hair and a beard to match. His patients love him. He loves his kids. He's still crazy about his wife after a lot of years together and I have no doubt that his dogs think he's pretty neat, too. He had been a PA almost since the position was first thought up and legitimized. (Some of you may not know what a PA is or the history of the profession, but bear with me and I'll get around to that later.) Mirno is a good-looking dude, although not as good-looking as me. Although he is a year or two younger than me, he almost immediately started referring to me as his kid brother.

The following week I showed up at his office as instructed. The office is in a five-story medical building next door to Lakes Region General Hospital, which owns the practice. Besides Mirno there were several nurses, a med tech, a receptionist, and two doctors. The doctor who had started the practice was about to leave to go work in Afghanistan. He wasn't a young guy either. It dawns on me that when some scumbag lawyer says in court that all doctors are just in it for the money, they ought to tread lightly.

Mirno and I worked out the details of scheduling and then immediately set to seeing patients. The way it worked was that the med tech would tell the patient that Mirno had a student with him and would ask if they minded if I came in and observed. Very few people refused, even though many of them were going to be dealing with some pretty intimate procedures and conversations. I found that women were much more amenable to my presence than men. I guess that over the years women get more accustomed to having their plumbing explored than men ever do. On that subject: certain of my male friends thought it was a big deal that I got to see women under pretty intimate conditions. Take it from me, there is nothing either fun, amusing or titillating about a pelvic exam. Certainly not for the person being examined, much less for the person doing the exam.

If I learned nothing else from Mirno I learned just how important bedside manner is. It became apparent pretty quickly why I'd been told that his patients loved him. He was serious when it was called for. He was always compassionate. He could deliver a gentle kick in the pants when appropriate. He was thorough. He was often funny. He respected everybody – that part was key. He didn't necessarily *like* everybody, but everyone was treated equally. Every medical practice has patients, and hopefully anyone reading this is not one of them, who are genuine pains in the ass. They show up constantly with vague symptoms that get explored six ways to Sunday when they're the only ones who think anything's wrong. Some people like the attention that they get. Others are looking for drugs, a subject that I will fully develop later. They take valuable time away from people who need real care. Only once did I see Mirno get aggravated. He was told that a certain patient had arrived for an appointment. His response: "Why the hell is he here again?" It was literally the only time that I saw him express anger. In the examining room, nobody was the wiser for Mirno's brief eruption.

I'm not going to give you the whole fifty hours here, just some snippets.

We walked into a room at 8:32 in the morning to a patient sitting on the examining table in his underwear. Mirno started laughing. The patient said, "What? What?" Mirno said, "The last thing I need to see first thing in the morning is you sitting there in your skivvies!" The patient laughed too. Mirno then got serious and said, "I'm going to give you another lecture about your blood/sugar and I know as usual you won't listen to me." The patient said, "I know, I know. The diabetes is going to kill me." Mirno started laughing again and said, "No. No, the smoking is going to kill you. The diabetes will just be a side show." We all had a chuckle. Mirno and I left the room and he immediately switched gears. We walked into the next room. An elderly man was sitting on the table. He was having trouble breathing. He had end stage lung cancer. Mirno said, "You know how I feel about you." The gentleman nodded. Mirno said, "The lab results aren't good. There's nothing left to do at this point. I'll be there for you and we'll deal with any pain that you have. Do you understand what I'm telling you?" The gentleman said, "I've had a good life. It's time for me to move on." Mirno took his hand and held it for half a minute. First off I thought, "What courage," but mostly I felt like I'd been hit in the chest with a baseball bat. I have no doubt that Mirno attended that man's funeral.

We had a patient who was having trouble with his prostate. He was a lawyer. Mirno said, "I'm going to check your prostate." (The dreaded rectal exam.) "Then I'm going to have Gerry check it. We both have serious issues with lawyers." The guy looked like he was choking on a bone. Then Mirno started laughing.

My time with Mirno went by quickly, and before I knew it, I was done. I thanked him profusely. He said, "Remember two things. Be confidant in what you do. You won't always be right but go with your gut feel. Secondly, treat everyone with the respect that you want from your own provider. Lastly, we don't take students around here for long periods of time. However, we're willing to make an exception in your case and take you for a clinical rotation, if you are lucky enough to get into the program." I left his office walking on cloud number nine.

The letter arrived. I had been accepted to the PA program at the Manchester, NH, campus of Massachusetts College of Pharmacy and Health Sciences. I would start on January 4, 2004, at 8:00 a.m. promptly. This time around I had not so much a feeling of jubilation as one of satisfaction. I had every confidence that I was finally heading down the right road. There wasn't time for much celebrating. I had an organic chem exam coming up and I was barely hanging onto a B average.

Now that I was in, there was the minor detail of how to pay for it. Tuition was thirty grand a year. With incidental expenses and the cost of travel every day plus lodging during my clinical year, I figured I was looking at seventy grand. I didn't want to take any student loans if I could help it. At my stage of the game, I'd just be working to pay off the loans for most of my upcoming career. I had already been provided with the answer.

Back when I was getting started with the nursing program, I had made contact with my ex-wife. I had explained to her that my situation had changed pretty dramatically, that I was no longer in the toy business, and that I was pursuing a career in medicine with all the inherent costs that entails. I wanted to know if she would consider a change in our alimony agreement that would allow me a little wiggle room. She said that she thought we could work something out and that she'd get back to me.

Several months later I was barely wiggling so I called her back. She didn't seem to have much recollection of our earlier conversation. I decided that the courts might be sympathetic, what with the unbeatable combination of my being the wonderful guy that I am and my entering this noble line of work. My lawyer was a slim, soft spoken, methodical guy. He thought it would be worth trying the legal route again, that my position might have "some credence." He had also recently taken up golf and was totally consumed by it. I think our conversation probably brought him a step closer to those Ping irons he had tried out.

My ex-wife's lawyer was auditioning for the part of Clarence Darrow in the remake of *Inherit The Wind*. He was a big guy with a shock of white hair who looked like he might have played a little college ball. He yelled a lot, waved papers in the air and got just the right amount of perspiration on his forehead. All in all, he worked himself into quite a lather.

My position: I'd been laboring in a dying business and all of my customers had been going broke, so there was no way I'd have been able to continue to make a living in that line of work. I kept the part about being completely burned out by it to myself. Clarence Darrow's position was that I was a lowlife bum who just wanted to sit around all day and not work for a living. He was so convincing I found myself starting to agree with him about the lowlife part.

At one point he waved a bunch of papers in the air (they could have been that morning's *Boston Globe* for all I knew) and said, "Look how much you're worth. You have a lot of nerve bringing this before the court." Well yes, I do have some nerve, but I replied, "Most of my net worth is in retirement accounts that I can't touch yet. The money that I need to live on and use for tuition is approaching the nickel and dime stage." He replied that the rules allowed me to withdraw money from those accounts to pay for tuition. He then glared at me and rested his case. I hadn't known that little part of the tax laws before, but I certainly filed it away now. On the way out of court I thanked the judge for his time. He sort of waved me out with a somewhat disgusted look on his face. I wondered if his sister was a nursing school instructor.

A few days later my lawyer called and said, "Bad news. The judge sided completely with your ex. Basically, you got screwed. Why don't we take it before the state Supreme Court?" He wanted a golf cart to go with the Pings. I decided to let it rest. Besides, the silver lining was that I now knew how to pay for school. I also hope that someday that judge comes into my hospital. He would be the only person in the history of medicine to ever get a rectal exam before having a splinter removed from his thumb.

As late fall turned into early winter, I started getting really pumped up to get onto the next stage. I got the grades I needed in microbiology and organic chemistry. I indulged in a great sigh of relief, then set to work seriously enjoying the month of December. I did quite a bit of skiing and patrolling but can only remember one incident. One brutally cold morning I was sent out to close a trail so the SnowCats could bring it back to perfection. The wind was whipping across the trail at about 30 miles an hour. Each time the cats came by I asked the drivers how much more time they needed. Each time they told me, "One more pass." They said that for about thirty- five minutes. All of a sudden I started feeling kind of strange and found that I was talking like someone with a dislocated jaw. I got on the radio and asked first aid top for a little relief. Curt Golder came back with, "Ah, K-42, maybe you ought to head down to first aid base." I got my skis on and kind of wobbled my way down there. When I got inside, Sharon Hannifan stuck two heat packs under my arms and gave me another one to hold on my face. Definitely the closest I've ever come to some type of hypothermic event.

# The PA Program

January 4, 2004, arrived with my alarm clock going nuts at 5:30 a.m. The early dawn had that cold, cold look to it. My wood stove had been cranking enough to keep the house at a toasty eighty degrees – eight hours ago. It was now fifty-four degrees and I couldn't get to the thermostat fast enough. My father, being the frugal fellow he is, had put a piece of duct tape on it at the seventy degree mark. I ripped it off and pushed the control to eighty-five. The gas burner let out a scream but proved to be up to the task.

As I got ready I noticed that I had no sense of nervousness or anxiety. Just excitement. I was finally about to start on the road to becoming a PA.

During the Vietnam war, most units had a corpsman, a soldier who had been trained in rudimentary as well as some advanced lifesaving techniques. If you got blown up in a rice paddy, this was the guy who was going to try to keep you stable until you could be brought back to a M.A.S.H. unit where the surgeons would attempt to piece you back together. I'd guess that many people alive today would tell you that they owed their lives to one of these folks. I'd also expect that a lot who didn't make it back took their last breath with a corpsman working feverishly over them. They were the precursor to the paramedic field as we know it today but they also were responsible for the field I was about to join. When the war was over there were a lot of extremely well-trained people who'd dealt with every eventuality that the carnage of war will bring. Some of them wanted to continue in medicine, but either felt they were too old for medical school or didn't have the financial resources to get there.

A forward thinking doctor at Duke University realized that these guys might be useful to society. He envisioned a class of medical providers who could work under the supervision of a doctor in poorly served, outlying areas of this country. The long and the short of it: there just weren't enough doctors to go around. The people in this field would have a good amount of medical training and would be able to perform many of the procedures a doctor does. If things got beyond their capabilities, a doctor could drive to them or provide an extensive explanation over the phone. While PAs would never be doctors, they'd certainly be better than no medical expertise at all.

That's a somewhat simplistic explanation of how it all got started. The profession has evolved way beyond its humble beginnings. You are now apt to deal with a PA or the nursing counterpart, a nurse practitioner or NP, in any hospital or medical practice in the country.

People often ask me what the difference is between what I do and a doctor does. I'll give you my take, which is most likely not going to be sanctioned by the American Academy of Physician Assistants. Doctors are PhDs in medicine. They are expected to know everything about everything. PAs and NPs have a Masters degree in medicine. We know a lot about some subjects and a little bit about everything. We are ethically bound to keep a doctor advised as to what we are doing with you, particularly if we run into something that we don't quite understand.

The job opportunities in this country exploded for both PAs and NPs when it was mandated that medical residents were no longer allowed to work one hundred plus hours a week. Residents are medical school grads – in fact, doctors who are still learning their craft. Like nursing students (but on a much higher scale), they functioned as slave labor working for long periods of time on two to three hours of sleep. They were starting to make mistakes. When Congress changed the rules, it opened the doors for PAs and NPs to step in as basically permanent residents.

At the same time I don't want to minimize the profession. Medical school, PA school and NP school are, like so many professions, just keys that open doors. A PA who's been in practice for ten years is probably going to be pretty damned good. In medicine you learn by doing. The difference from other professions is that you learn by doing on human beings.

\* \* \*

I walked in the door of the building that would be my campus for the next two years. It wasn't a fancy campus. The college consisted of two floors in a building that mainly housed the offices of Keyspan Energy. The main floor consisted of a large entry/waiting area, a small kitchenette and several very large lecture rooms. The decorating style was Early Stark. The basement consisted of faculty offices, a large simulation room much like the one from nursing school, and a computer room. Our library, an oversized closet, was still a work in process. I didn't care what it looked like. I was in PA school.

I noted some familiar faces from the day back in October when we had interviewed. I also noted that several people I'd talked to that day were not present. I asked somebody about one guy who I'd been sure would be accepted. He in fact had been accepted, but shortly after had been called up to serve in Iraq. That damned war got in the way for a lot of people. Ian Hamilton from ski patrol would be going; I hoped that his fiddle and guitar wouldn't get shot up while he was there. Several other ski patrollers were also called to serve. It dawned on me that if this many people I knew were going over there, then the scope of it all had to be huge.

We were all herded into one of the large lecture rooms and bumped into each other as we shuffled around looking to carve out our own space. Again, you'd probably keep whatever seat you started with. I settled on one in the back, in the far right corner, forgetting to take into consideration that slowly disappearing sight and hearing skills might create problems.

I surveyed the room. A quick count told me that there were twenty five of us. Ages ranged from early twenties to the fifty year old sitting in the back row, right hand corner. We seemed to be a representative microcosm of America today. Sixteen of the class were women. Two members were Russian. One of the guys was black and one was Indian. At least two of my class members were gay, and made no effort to hide it. Yep. Someone had put some thought into the makeup of this class.

The entire faculty marched in and stood lined up against the blackboards in the front. They were all PAs, except for a nurse who was the head of administration. Louise Lee was the head of the program. She had worked in emergency medicine and some office practices before finding her way to academia. She has a den mother quality but as I found out later, she could cut to the chase pretty quickly. Steve Steiner was an orthopedic PA with lots of operating room time. He reminded me of a young Mitch Miller. He had a quirky sense of humor that I grew to enjoy immensely. Patty Cousins had a background in family practice. She'd been a nurse prior to becoming a PA, and would leave at mid-year to help organize the PA profession in the U.K.

Gale Furey spoke last. She was the one I'd interviewed with in October. She didn't appear to have lost any cockiness. She exuded the military background that she'd come from. Her specialty was dermatology. She would be the point person for the first year students and was also to be my faculty advisor. She gave a no-nonsense speech that concluded with, "You will all struggle. We will throw so much information at you that it will be the intellectual equivalent of trying to take a drink from a fire hose. I am not here to be your friend. I am here to see that you succeed. I guarantee that you will all hate me by the end of this year."

We then took our first exam. It was on material that we'd been given to read over the holidays, on medical prefixes and suffixes. I got 100 but that material has never stayed with me. To this day I still find myself going to the medical dictionary to look up things like the difference between leukopenia and leukocytosis. Look it up yourself.

We were done by noontime. Well, shucks, I thought, this isn't going to be so bad. The rest of that first week was pretty manageable. Again, I am not going to give you every day of that year. I'll give you one year's worth of snippets.

On day one, the faculty had us go around the room and tell a little bit about ourselves. Just about everyone in the class had some sort of medical background – med techs, paramedics, etc. John Stallman was a PhD in organic chemistry. I figured he'd be the academic superstar of the class. Cheryl Elinsky was a physical therapist and had taught anatomy at several schools. That got her excused from most of our anatomy classes and exams. The professor basically said he didn't need someone sitting in the class who knew more than he did. I was also to learn later that she had swum around Manhattan and across the English Channel. You had to pull that stuff out of her. She was about five feet to my six feet plus. I started to refer to her as "Little Buddy," like Gilligan. I'm not sure if she liked that or not. It didn't matter. She couldn't reach high enough to punch me. Julia Skladchikova had been a doctor in her native Siberia. She struggled with English, which I believe was the main impediment to her attempting to get licensed as an MD in this country. Craig Roberts, a young black guy who had been a big-time swimmer in college, was from Bermuda. I asked him about the black swimmer part. It didn't seem to be a sport that attracted many blacks. He said, "I've been a lifeguard for as long as I can remember. And swimming is one of the quicker ways off the island."

When you write something like I'm doing, you like to get people's names into it – people like to read their names in print. I apologize to my classmates who I haven't mentioned. You had to have done something which was pertinent to the moment. A number of people I hung out with a lot won't ever get mentioned, like Stephen Cahill for instance. My apologies to you all.

* * *

The class seemed to be made up of a group of competitive over-achievers. The great thing is that this class meshed so well that the competitiveness never became an issue. Everyone was always available to everyone else for help, fun or support. I'm told that some of the other classes had problems along those lines.

The lectures began in earnest. Early on, our faculty members gave most of these. Then we started to get lectures from a long line of doctors. Adjunct professors, some we would only see once; others would come in for a series of lectures. They received a minimal fee and got credit for a certain amount of CME (continuing medical education) hours that all medical providers, PAs included, must maintain in order to stay licensed. They often used their lunch hours, days off, or came in before their office day began or after it had ended. Obviously there are people in medicine who feel it's important to pass what they know along to the next generation. We only had one or two doctors the whole year who acted like they really didn't want to be there. Since we students had to submit a review after every single lecture, I'd expect that some of the latter weren't invited back.

Not all of the lectures were scintillating. Not everyone in the world is adept at public speaking. Nor are all medical subjects fascinating to all people. Sometimes, though, we'd be surprised when we least expected it. One day in July an older doctor walked into the room at 5:00 p.m. His hair was rumpled. His suit was wrinkled. He didn't have the usual slick handouts we'd become accustomed to; we'd actually have to take notes like they did in the old days. He was going to give us two hours on diseases of the prostate and this was going to be torture. He stood in front of us nervously shuffling the few papers he'd brought with him. Two hours later, most of us were riveted to our chairs, hoping that he'd keep talking for another couple of hours.

The first of the great lecturers was right off the bat in January, Mike Carvalho, a pharmacologist – that is, a doctor of drugs. We usually had him at 7:30 or 8:00 in the morning. He was like a jolt of espresso at that hour. He never lectured for more than an hour and it was always a whirlwind of a lecture. What drugs to use. What pathway the drug took in the body and how it left. What drugs interacted with other drugs and food. What drugs never to use in certain instances. It went on and on. I loved it. I thought that, God forbid this PA thing didn't work out, maybe I'd try pharmacology next. I did great on his exams. He never tried to kill us and the exam questions were always right out of his lectures. Later in the year he got a standing ovation from the class when his series was done. Only one other doctor received one, earlier in the year.

* * *

At the end of January we had our White Coat Ceremony. We'd be receiving the half-length white coats that we would wear in all clinical and hospital environments. The half-length signifies student. Family was invited. My dad couldn't make it. He was off on one of his regular jaunts somewhere in the country. Christy took an afternoon off from work and was in the crowd. Gale Furey spoke. She said, "Nothing is given to you in medicine. We are making an exception this time. We are giving you these white coats. It signifies that you have been accepted into a very select fraternity: students of medicine. You will have to earn the full-length coat. You will then no longer be our students. You will be our colleagues." We then were called up individually and presented with our coat. It was an emotional moment. I looked for Christy in the crowd. She gave me a huge smile. Later she said, "Now I get it. You truly have entered into something special."

By the second week of February we were starting to settle into the routine and the feeling of drudgery started to settle in. Our days often went from eight to eight and we were getting tired. Plus some of us were starting to get a little lost. On any given day you were apt to get five lectures, all on disjointed subjects. Gale Furey marched in one morning and read us the riot act. She said that she was not at all impressed with this class and that we had better get our acts together pretty quickly. Most of all, she told us, she expected some people to drop the attitudes immediately.

She went on in that vein for a couple of minutes and then ended with, "I told you people that you would hate me by the end of the year." Since I can't keep my mouth shut, I added, "And it only took six weeks." She glared at me and marched out. I thought I heard her chuckle in the hall.

The faculty kept adding more and more work. Every time you got to a point where you couldn't handle anymore, you found out that you could. There'd be the occasional crying jag at lunch – some even came from the women in the class. The exams started to come in waves. Some days, we'd have three exams on three different subjects. Then the faculty told us that we would have to pick a topic, write a paper in a format suitable for medical publication, and present it to the class in PowerPoint format. This was the breaking point. We couldn't handle anymore. Several of us went to Louise and expressed those sentiments and asked if we couldn't just stick to learning medicine. We were told in no uncertain terms that we would get this done. "You are in a Masters Degree program and people in Masters Degree programs write a paper."

I was fascinated with gastrointestinal issues, maybe because I was always having problems with my own gastrointestinal tract. Imodium was my friend. I was thinking that I'd become a GI PA. People asked me, "Why do you want to deal with that yucky stuff?" I'd reply, "A lot goes on between when food goes in and comes out." My classmates started to refer to me as GI Gerry. I wrote my paper on the significant differences between colonoscopy and sigmoidoscopy in discovering colon cancer.

Dr. Gordan arrived one night in the spring. He had close cropped white hair, wire rim glasses and a signature bow tie, and spoke with what I would call a strong Teutonic accent. I remember turning to Eric Horton and saying, "Well, there won't be any fooling around with this guy." Eric agreed. Dr. Gordan lectured over a period of a few weeks on pulmonary function – that is, asthma, emphysema, lung cancer and arterial blood gas values, plus a whole bunch of other very complicated stuff. His accent caused us to have to ask him to repeat some things several times. Once we got used to the accent, though, he started to grow on us. He would get himself all worked up with enthusiasm and his signature word for emphasis was an "and" that came out as "unt." The "unt" was always said with great flourish. He became known as Dr. UNT. At the end of his series of lectures he got the standing O.

Pathology is basically the study of tissue, especially tissue that goes bad and causes disease. Path was taught to us by Dr. Tom Andrews and Dr. Jenny Duval. They were both coroners for the state. Dr. Andrews was very funny. Maybe you have to be to do his job. One day he was showing us slides of microscopic tissue from a tumor. He said, "Clearly this is tissue from a cancer of the prostate." We all thought, "Man, we have a lot to learn. This guy can tell that just by looking at this slide of protoplasm." I was marveling at his pure genius when he asked, "Do you know *how* I can tell that it is prostate tissue?" We considered his question for a moment. Finally he enlightened us: "It's written right here on the back of the slide."

The story on Dr. Andrews, which I never had the guts to ask, was that he'd been a pediatrician. Supposedly he had lost several of his little patients to things like crib death, all in one week, and couldn't take it anymore.

Dr. Duval was his opposite. She was calm, soft-spoken and rarely phased by much of anything. I asked her one day how she came to be a coroner. She said that while she really liked surgery, she was kind of shy and didn't like dealing with patients that much.

I saw my first autopsy, performed by Dr. Duval at Concord Hospital, where I had started my nursing training. The morgue, in the bowels of the hospital, was not too well marked. It took me a while to find it. I'm not sure what I expected it to look like. This one was an oversize version of a janitor's supply room – a very clean janitor, I hasten to add. People in this business are often said to have macabre senses of humor. The first thing I noted were all the cartoons on the walls that dealt with death and mad scientists. Next I noted several motorcycle helmets on a shelf. They all had cracks or holes right through them. A lot of folks in medicine refer to motorcycles as "donorcycles."

Dr. Duval walked in with a state trooper, whose job was to stand on a stepladder and take pictures. This case was officially a suicide, but foul play hadn't been ruled out. Our subject, a victim of hanging, had been having disagreements with her spouse. We pondered whether this might not be a cry for help and attention that got out of hand. I'm happy to tell you that, laying on a table in the morgue, you get treated with the same respect as if you were alive. The difference is that when this procedure is over, you have no secrets left to keep; the most minute detail has been noted and recorded. Since my first autopsy, I've always made sure to leave the house sporting clean fingernails and wearing clean underwear,.

Autopsy isn't for the squeamish. I'm no longer squeamish, but I didn't enjoy this procedure. I kept thinking, "Twelve hours ago you were alive and probably sitting at the kitchen table drinking beer. So sad."

There was a tremendous amount of cutting, but very little blood. As the abdomen was opened, the room filled with a sickly sweet smell. I got to know that smell quite well in surgical rotations but never found it again to be so strong, and I've never been able to get used to it. Organs are removed and weighed, and samples are taken for the lab. The contents of the stomach and intestines are noted. A vibrating buzz saw is employed at times which sends a mist of powdery bone around the room. A medical assistant accidentally dropped a section of skull on the floor. It rolled around like a dinner dish. She said, "Oops."

I was glad to have been allowed to witness this procedure and to have been allowed to participate. However mostly, I must admit, what I wanted was to go home and shower. It took several showers to feel normal again.

Once a week we had an afternoon in the clinical lab. The class was broken into three groups, each with a faculty member as an advisor. My advisor was Gale Furey. Actors and actresses were brought in and followed a script about whatever disease they were supposed to have that week, a lot like the Seinfeld episode where Kramer does the same thing. Our folks weren't as funny as Kramer, at least not intentionally. Sometimes though they'd forget the script or include material from the following week's script. It didn't happen often but when it did, it could really throw a student just learning the craft for a loop. You'd be thinking, "Aha. I know what this is." All of a sudden you didn't. Then Gale, who'd probably been sitting there half asleep would start rifling through her script and start mouthing to the actor, "You're off topic."

These exercises were not specifically about making a diagnosis. If you did diagnose it, so much the better; as the year went along we got pretty good at diagnosing and would often have the presenting problem figured out in a couple of minutes. However, at this point, our job was to learn how to interview a patient, sort out what was relevant, do a basic physical, and then form a differential of all of the things it might be. My nursing school training came in handy here. I was pretty comfortable with asking patients questions and performing a basic exam. I thought I was pretty good. Gale didn't. She made me a lot better. She had no problem with getting in my face like a drill sergeant, telling me to stop jumping to conclusions and take this seriously. Gale was considered the toughest advisor and some students were glad they didn't have to deal with her. Her style was perfect for me. She could be picky and sarcastic, but I knew that she was doing it for the right reasons. Later in the year it was decided that we would all rotate to other advisors. I begged her to keep me. She wouldn't.

Gale, as stated before, is a dermatology PA. She worked derm into every lecture, even if the subject was bones. One day someone said, "Gale, would you knock off the derm crap for a while?" She replied, "The skin is the most important organ. It keeps you from leaving all the squishy stuff inside all over the sidewalk."

We got into the middle of summer. We had lost two classmates. One had left about five weeks into the program, confiding to me, "I've never really had to work hard at anything in my life. This is too much for me. Plus I don't like the way they treat us. I'm going to go to nursing school." I didn't even begin to explain to him what I thought he might deal with there. I did call him at home and try to talk him into staying in our program. Tony Pellegrino, our class president, dropped out when his father died; he felt that the family needed him, and re-enrolled the following year. Mark Barros became our new Prez. He had played some hockey and was a hockey nut like I used to be. We talked about the great Bruins teams. His great Bruins teams came along about twenty years after my great Bruins teams. I just couldn't get away from this age thing.

August approached. This was becoming a relentless grind. We sat in lectures at seven at night and stared out the window as girls in shorts and flip flops walked by on the sidewalk. At least that's what I was staring at.

* * *

Remember the grouse back at the end of the first section? One morning around this time, my neighbor, Steve Reep, stopped at the top of my driveway on one of his morning walks. He said, "The grouse has met her demise." I replied, "You're kidding. What happened?" He reported that he and Schotzie, his Jack Russell terrier, had been working in his garage the day before, when the grouse had strutted around the corner and challenged Schotzie to a dust up – under a couple of vehicles, over a work bench and in behind his snow blower. The way Steve told it, the two were pretty evenly matched. In the end, Schotzie was sitting dazed in the corner with a mouth full of feathers and the grouse lay twitching on the ground. Steve said, "Well, at least I now have a great-looking feather for my Tyrolean hat.

I had grown to loathe that bird There was no sense of the loss of a worthy adversary, just good riddance to a first class nuisance. However, here is what I consider the strange part: "my" grouse had acquired a mate, a smaller, meeker version of herself. They looked not unlike a couple you might see strolling the aisles in Wal-Mart. I couldn't believe that anyone, especially another grouse, would find her attractive, but he was clearly quite fond of her.

A few days after the demise of Mrs. Grouse, I was standing in my family room, half paying attention to the evening news on T.V. but mostly miles away in thought. Suddenly there was a thwack on one of the big sliders right next to my head. I jumped back and looked out to see what appeared to be a hawk, staggering backwards on my deck. It took about three steps and dropped. I slid open the slider and went out to take a closer look. It was Mr. Grouse. I'm not sure if he committed suicide because of a broken heart, or maybe he somehow blamed me for the loss of his mate and was trying to take me out. In any case, this was decidedly too weird. I had a dusty, dog-eared copy of *The Exorcist* in my bookcase. I immediately threw it out. The next morning, the grouse still lay where he'd fallen. I put on work gloves, carried him into the woods and laid him on top of a big, flat boulder. May he rest in peace.

* * *

Christy and I started to struggle in our relationship. This program can take a toll on personal lives. Plus, I'm a pain in the ass to go out with. She and I were barely hanging on. I couldn't allow myself to get consumed by our issues. I had to stay totally focused on the task at hand. If she and I didn't make it, I'd have to mourn the loss later. Right now I had too much at stake to get sidetracked. I did tell her, though, that if I got through this and we were still together, I'd look for a job around southeastern Massachusetts where she lived. That, however, was a long time off. I didn't have to worry about leaving my beautiful woods yet. Besides, by the time I graduated, I honestly didn't think we'd be together anyway.

We actually got a vacation. They gave us a week off in August. I've never appreciated anything so much in my life. Christy and I took her kids to Niagara Falls. I was so glad that they were able to look at it with the same wonder that I had when I was their age. We also took a drive around Ontario and ended up at the St. Lawrence Seaway. It is hardly used anymore but we got to see a couple of big ships go through some of the locks. I also noted the names of all the little towns and identified them with the hockey heroes of my youth. It brought me back to a nostalgic time. Imagine, this little town is where Brad Park grew up. I kept that stuff to myself. None of this helped Christy and me. We took verbal jabs at each other the entire trip.

Labor Day went by, ushering in what was becoming my favorite time of year. Just think of all of the Patriots and Monday night football games that were coming up. I wouldn't get to watch too many of them – I'd be studying, but I made an exception for Boston College football. I hadn't gone there but had been a rabid fan ever since a guy from my home town named Fred Smerlas had played there. I didn't know him but I'd been around the Waltham boys' club when he came in to lift weights. He was the biggest guy I'd ever seen. The strongest, too. The guy he was working out with one day said to me, "You should see how much he can lift when his shoulder's not killing him." BC stunk at that time. Fred didn't, though. I think some day he may end up in the Pro Football Hall of Fame.

I'm not a super baseball fan, even though it was probably my best sport. I'd been a pitcher through Little League and high school. If I'd had any confidence I think I would have been pretty good. My father used to tell me, "Don't think too much. Just throw the damned ball." I always thought too much. Listening to my classmates it was evident that the Red Sox were going to make a run at the whole deal. I started sneaking peaks while studying during their games. As it got closer to October, the peeks started getting longer. We weren't, as I recall, allowed to skip any classes to watch games, but during certain games a secretary was allowed to come in on the half hour and give us quick rundowns. Our lecturers may have been doctors but right now, they too were Red Sox fans, first and foremost.

I know that I watched every playoff game against the Yankees. The only one that I remember involved a big brawl. Don Zimmer, the Yankee coach, had run out on the field and challenged Pedro Martinez. Pedro threw him down on the ground. The announcers took Pedro apart for beating up an old man. I had nothing against Don Zimmer but in this case I thought Pedro should have beaten the crap out of him. Once you cross those white lines…

What happened? The Sox were going to the World Series. It was pure theatre. The playoff games with the Yankees had been so exciting that I didn't bother even watching half of the series games. You just knew that the Sox would win. My classmate, Tracey Crossman, told me that baseball season had kept her 91-year-old great grandmother alive for a few extra months. I know that there were a lot of stories in the Boston area like that.

This incredible year was winding down fast. I could see the light at the end of the proverbial tunnel. I could take anything they could throw at me for another two months. Final exams arrived and they were brutal. I felt like the intellectual equivalent of the castaway on a desert isle. The clothes on my brain were all in tatters. I waved feebly at every ship that passed me by.

We had just one more little exercise to do before we could move forward into our clinical year, complete physical exams on several different people. Crash dummies would be used for the more intimate exams. We had to do the exams in appropriate order, call out what we were doing, make a correct diagnosis, and suggest an appropriate treatment. This would be an all- day affair.

My turn came and I was cranking right along. It's amazing how much you can learn in one year. Towards the end I was examining an actor who was supposed to be having problems that were bone-related. I got stuck. Steve Steiner was standing there with a clipboard. He said, "Take your time." The way he was tapping his foot didn't say, "Take a lot of time." I had lost my place and was getting flustered. I may have just imagined it, but the actor seemed to move her eyes in the general direction of where the problem was. Whether she did or not, I found my place and finished with a flourish.

Some of my younger classmates were now getting ready to go out and get bombed. I decided to go home and ski. Maybe I'd get bombed later.

I rode up the lift in early twilight. The lights were just coming on for night skiing. I wasn't patrolling; this skiing was just to blow off steam and relax. As I rode, I started to reflect on the past year. It was a really slow lift, so I had lots of time for reflection. I thought of how quickly a year that I never thought was going to end was now completed. I realized that a building that I'd grown to dislike going into every day had actually been a refuge. We'd spent an entire year shielded from the outside world in there, allowing us to focus exclusively on our goal. The birth process would now begin. I skied really hard for about two hours and then went home and lit the wood stove. I didn't get bombed, but I did get very relaxed.

*   *   *

Christy and I had split for a time, around Thanksgiving. She'd said that we were no longer what she envisioned, that she wanted to call it quits. If I hadn't been so wrapped up in school, I would have felt like the world had come to an end. As it was, it just sucked. The day before Thanksgiving, as we were leaving school for the brief holiday, I asked Cheryl Elinsky if I could talk to her in one of the offices. She followed me right in. I sat in a chair and she stood in front of me so we were eye to eye. I told her what was going on and started to cry. Not too many people get to see that side of me. She was wonderful. The combination of a good cry and her soothing words righted my sinking ship. I don't know why men don't have a good cry more often. It's very cathartic. I may suggest it to all of my future patients. Probably means I won't be providing medical service to the Marines anytime soon.

As Christmas approached Christy and I were trying to patch it up. We spent a lot of time together and talked more honestly and deeply than we had ever done before. By Christmas, 2004, all was right with the world.

# The PA Program
# Year Two: Rotations

During the second year of a PA program, as in the fourth year of medical school, students leave the classroom and go out into the clinical environment. You work with a primary doctor or PA, your "preceptor," and you work with any number of health care providers along the way. The student is now putting into practice all that was learned – or that rushed by – during the didactic year. You are still playing at medicine, but this is very serious play. You don't make the final decisions on patients, nor do you do anything without the approval of your preceptor.

At the same time, you quickly come to realize that these pros expect more of you than just staring at them wide-eyed, expecting them to tell you what to do. Once they develop a comfort level with you, they allow you a certain amount of freedom to work autonomously. It's still their ass on the line, so nobody's going to run off and do some quick brain surgery or anything, but you start to see a lot of patients on your own. When you're done and have made a quick presentation to the preceptor, you both go back into the room and the preceptor repeats part of the exam. The pro then tells you why you were right or wrong. As with my shadowing of Mirno Pasquali, patients are told that a student will be involved unless they would prefer to just see the primary care person. Very few people refused to see me over the course of the year. A lot of older people seemed to enjoy the added attention, and since they're most often the ones with ailments, it works well for the student, too. The difference between this and just shadowing is that now the student is doing the exam and some of the procedures.

My year would consist of five- or six-week rotations in Psychiatry, Family Medicine, Surgery, Internal Medicine, Emergency Medicine, Family Medicine (again), Pediatrics, Women's Health and an elective rotation.

## Psychiatry

I started on January 9, 2005, in psych. My preceptor was one of the few PAs in northern New England who practiced in this specialty; Gale Furey told me that she only took one student a year, so I should act like I was into psych, even if I wasn't. I didn't have to act. I like psych.

My preceptor was a wiry little black woman named Jumes Babatunde. She had great big eyes made bigger by great big glasses. She had a musical accent reminiscent of the Rasta men of Jamaica. She was actually, if memory serves me correctly, from Nigeria. She'd been trained as a nurse in her native country and then moved to the U.S. after getting married. She went back to school in Boston to become a PA and fell in love with psychiatry. She was now raising three kids on her own. The two older ones were in various stages of Ivy League educations. The younger one, the one she referred to as the smartest of them all, was already talking about Harvard.

She explained that I would just observe her for the first day and then she would bring me into things at a pace she felt that I was up to. By about the fourth day, she was letting me do most of the interaction with patients. She also had me start to suggest appropriate medications, write prescriptions and suggest follow-up therapy and visits, all of this under her watchful eye as she sat across from me and her patient.

This practice was not like the psych practices you see in the movies. No Woody Allen came in to lie on the couch for four hundred bucks an hour. Some of these people were very sick and would not have been able to function without the wonders of modern pharmacology. Some could also be aggressive, at which point this little Nigerian lady turned into one tough cookie. She'd get right into someone's face and say, "Get a greep on yourself, mon. I am not your problem. I am trying to help you find a solution." There were a few times when I felt that we were one step from violence. It never seemed to phase her.

For the most part, Jumes maintained a professional and detached demeanor. At other times, though, she'd let down and have a heart to heart with patients, and the empathy would pour out. There was never pity in her voice – sympathy yes, but she left no doubt that the patient was going to have to dig him or herself out with her support.

One day she had me work with the psychiatrist who was, in essence, her boss; she practiced under the auspices of his license. I met him at his office on a very cold morning and we set out to visit several nursing homes. He was like no doctor I'd ever met. A great big guy, he was easy going and quick witted. He was also quick to laugh at other people's humor. After about ten minutes together, I felt like I'd known him for a long time. I asked him about his family. He said, "I recently lost my life partner to a rare cancer. I'm trying to get over it. I'm not sure that I ever will." I took a deep breath. I didn't know what to say. Finally I said, "Maybe you're not supposed to get over it." Over the course of that day we shared a few things with each other that strangers and preceptor/students probably don't. I felt like I had made a connection with this man, even if it was only over the course of one day. It was unlikely that I would ever see him again.

We visited nursing homes. One of them had been a mental institution, back in the days when we referred to them as such. It still had that institutional feel to it and wasn't a particularly comfortable place to be. It had the smell of an institution and the sounds of commotion and people crying, the wailing of people with dementia. After just a little while, all of that fell into the background. I started getting into the whole thing and watching this doc interact with patients and staff. We then went into a locked ward. It seems odd to be talking about elderly people in a lockdown situation, but apparently some of these folks were capable of taking quite a run at you. We went to the nurses' station and wrote a number of orders and follow-up notes.

While I was waiting to leave, I was standing against the wall next to a sweet looking elderly woman who was sitting in a wheel chair. She was a tiny little thing and had a somewhat vacant smile on her face. A nurse hustled by and in passing said to me, "I'd move away from her just a bit. She'll grab your balls if she gets the opportunity." I took a giant step to the left and thanked the nurse profusely.

On the ride back we talked about Alzheimer's disease. It doesn't just effect the elderly. I'd seen two people in their fifties in rapid decline. One of them had been a doctor who'd started forgetting how to use some of the basic medical instruments in his office. Many of these people had devoted family and spouses who visited every day. For those of you who are lucky enough not to have first hand experience with the disease, imagine what it would be like if the person you love the most in your world started to no longer recognize you. It is easily, painfully, one of the most devastating disease that we deal with, not so much for the patients, but for their families.

This rotation went by quickly. Jumes gave me an excellent evaluation that ended with her writing that she felt that I was going to be a strong PA. I told her that I probably wouldn't end up in psychiatry, but wouldn't mind working in the field if that's what I was led to. I was starting to have a spiritual feeling – and I'm not an overly spiritual guy – that there was a plan in place for me and I had best just go where it led me.

As advanced as we become as a society I don't believe that mental illness will ever lose the stigma that goes with it. I don't know why. If you have diabetes it is accepted – lots of people have it. If you have bipolar disease you are apt to act in ways that are considered inappropriate. As many people probably have mental illnesses as have diabetes. Some of them can hide it. Many are able to function in society because of the wonderful drugs now available. I believe these drugs do more to improve people's lives than most of the drugs used to treat cancer. The mentally ill are all around you. They may be your neighbor, your mailman, or the person that teaches your kids. In most cases, you'll never know it. They work very hard to function from one day to the next. God love them.

# Family Medicine

My next rotation was in family medicine. Maybe Mirno had forgotten the part about taking me on again but I hadn't. The school had approved a five week rotation at New England Family Health where he practices. I felt like I was going home. The office is about nine minutes from my house and the building also houses my own doctor's practice, so I guess I *was* kind of home. As much as I had enjoyed psych, I'd been concerned that my medical skills would get rusty from disuse. Not to worry. It took about twenty minutes to shake the dust off.

I got to the office before Mirno and renewed acquaintances with the staff. I then went and checked the box of donuts and was told that unless I really wanted to piss Mirno off, I should leave the chocolate covered ones alone. He strolled in a few minutes later, saw me, rolled his eyes to the heavens and said, "What did I do to deserve this?" I replied, "Pick on someone your own size." He said, "You're bigger than me." I shot back, "I mean intellectually." He said, "Let's get going. You watch me for a day, then we'll let you start to get your feet wet."

I know that I loved this rotation. I was allowed to see a ton of patients. I just can't recall much of it. It was early in the year and I've seen a couple of thousand people since. So, a few more snippets.

Mirno and I went next door to the hospital to do rounds. We stopped in the room of someone who had lung cancer and was in the end stage of life. The person would take some breaths and then stop breathing. Mirno grabbed me by the arm and said, "Oh my God, this person is going to die right in front of you." I replied, "Mirno, that's just Cheyne-Stokes breathing." This often takes place at the end of life when the body is shutting down systematically. He replied, "At least you learned something in the past year."

Mirno was telling me about his early days as a PA. Having joined the Peace Corps, he was in Africa taking care of our volunteers there. I asked him if he liked it. He said, "Well, I met my wife there. She was a nurse in a village. I built her an outhouse; she's been eternally grateful ever since." He told me that one day he was riding his Vespa motor scooter along a dirt road on his way to see the recipient of the outhouse. A black mamba, the deadliest snake in the world, slithered out onto the path. They are also very fast and tend to grumpy dispositions. Mirno was too close to swerve or stop, leaving him no choice but to run the snake over. Looking back to make sure the snake wasn't chasing him, he says that it had reared up to about four feet in 'height' and was looking down the road at him as if to say, "What the hell did you do that for?"

One day Mirno was performing a physical on a middle-aged guy. He said to me, "This fellow has a perfect prostate." He asked the patient if I could check his prostate. The patient was none too thrilled about another finger up his butt, but

I guess in the interest of furthering medical education, he agreed. I slipped on a glove and slathered on copious amounts of Surgilube. I did the exam as quickly as I could. I felt nothing. Typically what you are looking for is as follows: a prostate gland feels like the area in your palm just above your thumb. Push your thumb towards your little finger. You want to feel a smaller version of that with two symmetrical sides, basically the size of a walnut. If either of the sides of the walnut has a hard pea in it, it calls for additional follow-up. Mirno asked, "Did you get it?" I replied, "Yup." Later in his office I told him, "Mirno, I couldn't feel anything." He said, "Just as I suspected. You can't tell the difference between your elbow and anybody's ass."

Mirno did a lot of minor surgical procedures. If someone had a funky looking freckle that was a concern, Mirno took it off, often resulting in the need for a suture or two. This was the part of my game that I was most concerned about. I was just not good at it. The disconnect: if you are going to work in the medical profession you have to be able to sew. For me it was the same as doing knots on ski patrol. I wasn't good at it, but you just needed to master a couple of them.

I knew I was bad at this. Before I had left school in December I had asked Steve Steiner to work with me. He was happy to oblige. He brought out the surgical tray and a pig's leg and we went to work. He took me through the process several times. Each time I attempted to repeat what he was showing me. After a while I was starting to do a little better. He said, "You're getting it. It's all about practice." I still didn't feel good about my skills. Mirno let me make numerous tries. Sometimes I got it, but more often than not he would have to take over. My hands would be shaking too much. I knew I had to get over this. There is so much suturing in medicine that you just can't be constantly looking around for someone to step in for you. It needs to be as second nature as zipping up your coat.

A woman came into the office one day looking just about as sick as I've ever seen. In medicine you have to be able to spot sick and not sick. I was as good at discerning sick as I was bad at sewing. She and her husband had been in Florida for the winter when she started to feel kind of crappy. She got worse, and told her husband to drive her back to New Hampshire. The way she was feeling, she wanted to see no one but Mirno. She got much worse in the Carolinas. By the time I saw her she was looking like death. I'd never seen someone who looked as sick as this lady. She was green. She couldn't breathe. She was vomiting every twenty minutes. She brought out all the empathy in me. I felt terrible for her. I did a physical and, while doing so, gave her the royal treatment. After a while, Mirno came in, held her hand for a bit and then started writing a laundry list of prescriptions. He told her to come back in four days.

She came back. She was alive, and she was a different person. She was ready to go back to Florida. She said, "I have never received treatment like you two gave me from any doctors in my life. You were both wonderful to me. You are like

Batman and Robin." After she'd left, Mirno said, "You just got you first psychological pay check. It makes it all worthwhile." He added, "Just don't confuse who's Batman and who's Robin."

This rotation was winding down. I would have been happy if my graduation had been tomorrow and I'd been hired to work in this office with people that I'd gotten to know pretty well. I'd come to think that working in a family practice setting was what I was probably going to look for. I was comfortable in that area of medicine and I thought that it offered me all the challenge I'd need. I was getting better at this. My history taking and physicals were now becoming second nature and very consistent in their order. I still wasn't right about every diagnosis. Often I'd give Mirno the run down and then suggest what I thought we were dealing with. He'd reply, "That's interesting. I hadn't thought of that." Usually he wouldn't think of it again, either. Sometimes though he'd say that my idea was worth exploring "a little more."

My next rotation was surgery, and I wasn't looking forward to it at all. Surgery is ripe with ritual and protocol. I don't like ritual and protocol. You have to scrub up and get the gown and gloves on appropriately and you have to keep your hands above your waist. There are certain things you can touch and certain things you can't. God forbid you turn your back on the instruments while within five feet of them. There were just too many opportunities for a klutz like me to screw up. I told Mirno all of this. His advice: "Just get through it. Not all of us are cut out to be surgeons." He related a story of how he struggled in his surgical rotation.

Mirno gave me a really good review. He shook my hand, wished me luck, and said, " Always protect yourself."

# Surgery

Most people in medicine don't work what would be considered normal hours. Surgeons really don't. I was to meet the new team at 6:30 a.m. for rounds. My rotation was at Caritas Hospital in Brockton, Mass., and I'd be staying with Christy for this rotation. As if seeing how I'd do as a surgeon wasn't challenge enough, we'd see how we did together living like a real couple, to boot.

The day before the rotation started was Easter. I scrambled to find a church in her area and just made it to Mass. As is always the case on Easter, it was jammed. I go to church most Sundays. I figured that, with this next rotation coming up, this was no time to risk pissing God off by missing Easter Mass. Afterwards I went with Christy and her kids to an Easter brunch, a tradition of hers honoring her mother who'd died of lung cancer a few years before. Christys' daughter, Kayla, age seven, and her son, Anthony, age nine, are normal kids. They act like kids. My problem is that sometimes I expect them to act like they're twenty-five. I haven't yet learned to keep my mouth shut with Christy when they act in ways I disapprove of. My mouth has always gotten me into trouble.

I got up at 4:30 a.m. to get ready to wrestle with surgery. Down to her basement, I threw around some old dumbells I'd brought with me, and was on the road by 5:55. The hospital was only twenty minutes away but I sure as hell wasn't going to be late. I got there about 6:15 and found my way to the med/surg floor where I met a first year resident named Vic, who looked like he had already been up for quite a while. He had been. He was responsible for presenting patients to the team. The white coats started to arrive. My preceptor was Dr. Richard Paulson. He was supposed to be about my age but looked about ten years younger. He looked a little like the Sundance Kid, actually, if the Kid had had salt and pepper hair. Next came Dr. Peter Augustinos, a big guy with jet black hair. He was two years out of residency and marched down the hall hunched over, with his hands jammed deep into the pockets of his coat. Last came Dr. Chris Corey, who was also supposed to be my age, and also didn't look it. He had a wispy moustache that with a little more trimming would have looked like an Errol Flynn special. He looked like nothing in the world had ever bothered him. The head resident, Sean Doherty, was in his sixth or seventh year. Surgeons do much longer residencies than other docs. It wasn't long before Dr. Corey started to refer to Sean and me as "The Flying Doherty Brothers." Three other residents, some pharmacy students, and a pharmacologist rounded out the team.

Residents are in fact doctors. They are not in their own practice yet but are honing the craft in whatever specialty they've chosen. This is their apprentice-ship. They provide the last word in slave labor and handle a lot of the medicine in any teaching hospital. Sean, the head resident, started firing questions at Vic. The docs all joined in. I felt like they were beating the crap out of him and that they were enjoying it immensely. I immediately felt defensive for him. Every morning started like this. No one considered it any big deal. It was all part of learning to be a surgeon.

After they were done chewing on Vic, Dr Paulson told me to join him. That meant having a conversation on the gallop. I would learn that he never stayed in one place very long, except of course in the operating room. Other than that, he was always on his way to someplace. He was the Chief of Surgery at the hospital so I guess he had to take a lot of meetings. He told me I could be involved in any procedures that I wanted and with whichever doctors that I wanted. They had one more doc in the practice, Dr. Richard Grotz. Dr. Paulson wanted me to get the full flavor of surgery and to see as many different procedures as possible. He also told me that I was welcome to go in with surgeons from other practices. Then he was gone down a side stairwell. It was now 7:10 a.m.

I found my way to the operating room lounge. No one was there so I looked around a little bit and then plopped on an overstuffed couch. A nurse walked in, a woman with beautiful eyes and a vivacious demeanor. She asked if I was the new student. I said that I was indeed. She said, "I'm Gail." Dr. Corey often referred to her as the hottest looking grandma in southeastern Mass.

She said, "Go into the locker room and get some scrubs on. I'll show you around and show you how to scrub up and gown." You spend all of your time in scrubs in surgery so from then on, every day started in the locker room with a change from street clothes into scrubs. There were piles of them, supposedly sorted by size, at the back of the room on a series of long shelves. At the end of the day, scrubs were thrown into a big laundry bin. I couldn't always find my size. Some days, I felt like I was walking around in a full length Speedo. With clothes that you might be wearing for twelve or thirteen hours, big and loose was definitely the preferred option.

I came out of the locker room and she said, "Go back in and get some shoe covers and a hair net." I slid the shoe covers on and found one of the paper and cloth hats that tied in the back. It made my ears stick out.

We then headed down the hall to the operating theatre. She pressed a button on the wall that opened the hydraulic doors. We went through. We were still in the same hall, but now you had operating rooms on both sides, eight or ten of them. Certain procedures were done in certain rooms; you learned pretty quickly where you were headed. You could look through picture windows into each room and some of them already had activity going on. Each room had a big trough of a sink next to it, with three faucets and a number of foot peddles beneath. From here on out you didn't touch anything that wasn't sterile.

They had shown us back in school how to scrub for surgery and I remembered enough of it so that Gail could say, "Looks like you have washing your hands under control." The idea is to not touch anything but water. You step on one pedal to get soap, another for cold water and another one for hot water. That part I never got right. I always got cold water. Sterile brushes in plastic wrappers dispense from above the sink. If you are going into surgery, the last non-sterile thing that you'll touch is the wrapper. You then hold your arms and hands under the faucet with your hands upwards. You want the water to drain down to your elbows. You start with your fingernails. You are supposed to spend one minute on each finger and nail, though I never saw anyone who took that much time. You then wash each hand, wrist, and arm to the elbows. When you're done you hold your arms up and away from your body. You then back through the door to the O.R. Your back is not considered sterile, therefore you have to watch how close you are in proximity to the sterile surgical field when turning around. If the sterile field is ever broken, then the patient has to be redraped and people have to go, scrub again and regown. You can imagine how pleased they'd be if some bonehead PA student caused that to happen.

At this point you already have on the surgical mask that ties around your head; that went on before scrubbing. The next step: someone holds up the gown for you to walk into, making sure you don't touch the outside of it. Next, someone holds out the sterile gloves, stretched to make it easier to slide your hands into them. These you jam your hands into with a flourish. After about a week of this, one of the operating room techs said to me, "You're getting better at this." I was quite pleased with the complement. She continued, "You're actually starting to get the right fingers in the right holes on the first try." The last step: you hold a sterile tab on the gown ties, spin around once to bring the ties around you, and tie the gown in front. If you are in six procedures during the course of a day, you will go through all of that six times.

When Gail was through with all of this, I headed back out to the general area. Around a corner was a large washable marker board that listed what procedures would be done at which time, in which room, and by which surgeon. It also listed which resident would be the first assist and who the other personnel in the room would be. Your average procedure was going to be staffed, in addition to the surgery team, by an anesthesiologist, a tech who prepared the equipment and handed it to the table, and a couple of circulating nurses who'd come in and out of the room bringing whatever else might be needed during the surgery. They also kept track of what was used for the purpose of billing. Everyone but the anesthesiologist and the circulating nurses were considered part of the sterile field.

I saw that none of the surgeons on my team had anything scheduled before 9:30. Something started at 8:00; I asked that surgeon if I could scrub in. He said, "Why not. The more the merrier." He had what sounded like a Russian accent. We scrubbed together. He told me that he'd gone to medical school in Slovakia and then done it all over again at N.Y.U. At this point I didn't know a good surgeon from a bad one but I could spot cocky. This guy was cocky. After going through the gowning procedure he was ready to go. He would be removing a parathyroid gland, the little lump that's attached to the bigger lump that is your thyroid gland. This part of the anatomy can be found just outside of your Adam's apple.

The patient was out cold. I was standing just off to the side of the table with my hands folded against my chest. I was trying to stay out of the way and be unobtrusive. He looked at me and said, "There's no place for shyness in an O.R. Get in here and put your hands on top of the patient until I tell you to do something." He had the resident do most of the initial cutting. He stepped in once the underlying anatomy was exposed, found what he believed to be the offending parathyroid, and removed it.

In real life, your parts don't come labeled like in the anatomy books. A lot of things look to be pretty much the same. You better know the difference. A little nick in the wrong place can spell huge trouble. The resident closed and sewed layers on her way out. I had actually gotten to participate. I think the doctor was mostly trying to keep my hands busy. The resident told me later that this doc was considered to be a really good surgeon and that residents liked him because he let them do a lot.

I got out of the procedure in time to join Dr. Corey who was already scrubbing for his first operation of the day. It was to be a carotid endarterectomy. Your carotid arteries carry blood to your brain. If one gets gunked up, you are at increased risk for a stroke. If it gets real gunked up, a portion can be removed and replaced with a graft.

Dr. Corey and I backed into the O.R. He is not one of those surgeons who believes that the O.R. is as sacred as a cathedral sanctuary. He likes chatter, and he especially likes it when he's doing most of the chattering. He tells jokes that sixth grade boys might consider dirty, though they're nothing compared to the stuff you're apt to hear from older guys. Most operating rooms are not exactly bastions of political correctness.

Dr. Corey let me make the initial incision. He had instructed me to use a light touch, "about the amount of pressure you would use to write your name so that it would go through two pieces of paper." I made a straight incision about 2.5 inches in length. A thin streak of blood followed my cut.

Surgery these days is a fairly bloodless procedure for the most part. Scalpels are used for some of the cutting still, but most is done with an electrical cauterizing tool called a 'bove.' The bove creates a fair amount of acrid smoke which gets sucked up by the ever-present suction tube. During my surgical stint I did a lot of this kind of thing. I also spent hours pulling on different sized retractors. After a while your arm goes numb. You have to constantly shift around just to stay comfortable. A student the previous year had problems with this aspect of things. Dr. Corey had finally gotten exasperated with him and asked, "What? Are you paralyzed or something?" It turned out that due to an accident the student had nerve damage in his arm; he was, in fact, somewhat paralyzed.

Dr. Corey took over. Carefully dissecting layers and moving muscle and nerves gently out of the way, he finally exposed the carotid artery and started clamping around where he would be cutting. There are always several people in close proximity around an operating table. It's not the optimal place for big bodies, but we had several of them squeezed in around this one. I was to Dr. Corey's right, at the level of the patient's head. Dr. Corey was neck high. I was trying to (a) stay out of his way and at the same time (b) keep pressure on the retractor to keep the wound open. This involved some fairly advanced-level contortions.

So Dr. Corey says "This skunk walks into a bar..." At this point one of the clamps holding the artery let go and blood started squirting as if from a super soaker. In three seconds, those of us in close proximity were covered in it. The surgical wound filled up like a pot hole in a spring downpour. Dr. Corey was no longer amused or amusing. He was deadly serious. One of the technicians called out that both blood pressure and oxygen levels in the brain were dropping. I stuck my thumb into the wound trying to occlude wherever the blood was coming from. Sean Doherty on the other side of the table stuck the suction tube in but it was filling up as fast as he was suctioning it out. Dr. Corey pushed me out of the way and stuck both of his thumbs into the wound. At this point an operating room tech decided it was a good time to start collecting instruments and pushed her way into the middle of things. Dr. Corey hissed, "Get out of my face. I'm not kidding you." He glared at her. The bleeding stopped and the clamp was replaced. After another minute or so, things stabilized. Dr. Corey said, "So anyway, this skunk walks into a bar and..."

I thought to myself, "God. I love this." I decided at that moment that I wanted to be a surgical PA.

The old saying about surgeons is that their philosophy of medicine can be summed up in one phrase: "to cut is to cure." One day I asked Dr. Augustinos if he thought that unfair. He said, "I don't know any surgeons who do procedures that aren't warranted. I also believe that in a disease like cancer, the outcome is often better after surgery than after drugs." After enough experience, I found myself agreeing with him. However, I got the flip side of that equation one day when I asked a surgeon why we were doing a particular procedure. He said, "Because I've got two kids in medical school. Any other questions?" He was kidding but anyone hearing that remark would have said, "See, I told you they do that."

What surgeons really do is sew. They are all good at it, but some are true artists. They can get into the tiniest space with a little needle and the finest thread and leave you better off than with the original parts that came under manufacturer's warranty. One such artist was a doctor at this hospital who was basically retired, though he still came to meetings and hung around because I think he simply couldn't get the environment out of his system. Someone asked him once how he had learned to sew like he did. He said, "It all started on the Thanksgiving when I was nine years old. My mother let me sew up the turkey's ass. The rest is history!"

I started to regularly scrub in with Dr. Grotz. He was more or less the abdominal specialist. Like the rest of these guys he didn't look his age; he had that pink-faced, recently-scrubbed look that radiates health. I knew that he got up every day at 4:00 a.m. to run his five miles. Still, there had to be more to why these guys all seemed so healthy. It couldn't be because of sleep – none of them did much of that. It couldn't be diet – they subsisted on stale donuts and saltine crackers that served as barges for peanut butter. I believe those food groups have been ruled out as youth enhancers. I decided that it had to be all that pure oxygen that gets pumped into the operating rooms.

Outwardly Dr. Grotz was the most serious appearing of the docs in the group. He didn't tolerate much nonsense and was quick to take over if a resident or a student started to fumble. On the other hand, he loved rock and roll circa the summer of 1969. He liked it blaring in the O.R. when he backed in. I often found myself wondering, as the opening riff to "The Last Time" by the Stones vibrated through the room, if the patient mightn't just get up and start shucking and jiving around the place.

As a student of medicine you're expected to answer questions about the subject whenever anyone feels like grilling you. It is called pimping. Some doctors are relentless at it and it definitely becomes tiring for the student. Often, the more you answer correctly, the more you get pimped. That's never been one of my problems. Dr. Grotz pimped about music. After a while it became evident that I knew more about subjects like Grace Slick and Steely Dan than he did. I started pimping him. He loved it. He'd say, "I love having you in my operating room." I'd reply, "I don't know why. My skills are lousy." He'd say, "But, man, you know your music." He also told me that I pulled the best retractor that he could ever recall. He never said anything about my sewing. He was known to tap his foot impatiently while I was doing it.

With Dr. Grotz I also witnessed some of the more gruesome procedures that surgery has to offer. Abdominal surgery can often involve very large incisions where a whole bunch of your parts get pulled out, sorted through and cut out. Then the rest gets sort of stuffed back in and patted around to smooth things out. Based on the way we brutalized the human anatomy during these procedures I expected to see patients writhing on their beds, screaming for morphine. It never failed to amaze me that, as we would do rounds the next day, most of his patients would say that they felt pretty good. Never underestimate the resilience of the human body.

As I've stated, surgeons aren't clock watchers. By the end of my first week I'd logged fifty-eight hours in the hospital, nothing by some standards but I was ready for a weekend off. On Friday afternoon around 4:00 p.m., I backed in to the O.R. with Dr. Corey. We were going to do a procedure that should have lasted until about 6:30. Unfortunately the patient was elderly and frail, and had also had a number of prior surgeries, which can really complicate things. From the start nothing went right. At about 6:15 Dr. Corey said to a nurse, "See if Dr. Grotz is still here." A little while later Dr. Grotz walked in wearing street clothes and holding a surgical mask over his face. Dr. Corey asked, "Are you doing anything?" Dr. Grotz replied, "I'm supposed to be at my kid's soccer banquet in twenty minutes. You need help?" Dr. Corey said, "Yeah. I could use another set of hands." Dr. Grotz came back in five minutes later, scrubbed and gowned. At 7:30 Dr. Augustinos called in on the intercom and asked them if they needed help. Dr. Corey broadcast, "Peter, go home to your new wife." Dr. Augustinos seemed let down that he wasn't invited to the party. At 9:30 Dr. Corey was sitting on a stool with his arms held against his chest. He looked tired and frazzled, at least from what I could see of him behind his surgical mask and magnifying lenses. He said to Dr. Grotz, but mostly to himself, "All right, let's go over this." They reviewed what they had done so far. They talked about where they wanted to get to and why they were stuck. Back to the table. At 11:00 Dr. Corey looked across the table at me and said, "You're a student. I want you to go home and enjoy the weekend." There's an unwritten rule in medicine: you finish what you start. I downplayed my hypocrisy and skeedaddled out of there as fast as my tired legs would carry me. I asked him the following week what time they'd gotten done. He said, "About 1:30." Very glamorous life these surgeons lead.

I was in on a procedure one morning where one of the residents was doing most of it. He worked fast. He asked the O.R. tech for an instrument which wasn't immediately forthcoming. The resident asked again, a bit impatiently. The tech said, "Fuck off. Can't you see I'm busy?" I almost swallowed my tongue. I'd come to view these residents as gods. The resident said nothing and the procedure continued. These folks work together on a regular basis and develop a tremendous sense of familiarity. Some of them don't necessarily love each other, but they all work in unison for the good of the patient. However, each person in the O.R. has a place in the hierarchy. No one in the O.R. puts the surgeons on the same pedestal that I had them on.

People working around the operating table occasionally get "stuck" with an instrument – it qualifies as an occupational hazard. Because of the serious blood-borne diseases that are now a part of life, there's an initial feeling of dread on the part of the 'stickee.' One day we were doing a kidney removal and a resident named Hasni got stuck with an instrument that looked like a two-inch pitchfork, used to hold tissue back. He yelped and spun away from the table. His finger bled through the surgical glove. He was told to go to the emergency department immediately for a blood test and a shot. He changed gloves and said that he would finish the procedure. Afterwards I accompanied him for moral support.

He was now a patient, and he didn't like it one bit. A nurse came in to draw blood. Hasni turned white. He said, "I think I'm going to pass out." I held him by the shoulders but I told him nonstop what a baby he was. He laughed but he got a little sweaty. The nurse asked him if he'd prefer to lie down. He replied, shrugging his head at me, "What I'd really prefer is that he be the one who gets stuck." I knew how he felt. I have no problem at all in dealing with your blood, but I'm still not thrilled about seeing my own.

When you've witnessed the same surgical procedure enough times, you start to think that you could perform it yourself. There were several procedures at this point that I probably could have gotten through in decent fashion. The difference is that I would always have had the surgeon there like a big brother looking over my shoulder. The defining moment is when things go bad, as they often do.

That's when you want the years of experience with the 'I've seen it all' attitude behind it. It's comparable to when you are flying along at 35,000 feet and the voice from the cockpit says, "We have a little problem here but nothing to worry about." You want that voice to sound like it has *at least* forty years of flying time behind it.

I figured out the time pattern on procedures. I knew that if I went into one at 3:30, I probably wouldn't be out in time to get into the one starting at 5:30. This resulted in weeks where I clocked forty-five hours rather than fifty-eight hours. For the balance of this rotation, things were a breeze.

I got a pretty good evaluation from Dr. Paulson. He did write that I needed to improve my sewing if I wanted to continue in surgery. If he wasn't such nice a guy it would have read, "Needs to learn to sew if he has any hope of continuing in medicine!"

On the personal side, Christy and I weren't getting along so well living as a couple. We argued about everything. By the end of the rotation we were barely speaking, not unlike some married couples I know... She couldn't see why, if I loved what I was doing, I should be coming home exhausted and grumpy. What she didn't see was that even though I did love it, not all of it came naturally to me, and that I can put tremendous pressure on myself. We broke up on the last day of the rotation. I would start my next rotation in a real funk.

# Internal Medicine

My next rotation was to be Internal Medicine, serving at the Veterans Hospital in Manchester, NH. Back home. I figured that after surgery, this was going to be a vacation. I may have been a little off on that. I had two preceptors who were both PAs, Joe Rivet and Dan O'Brien. They were also recent graduates of my program. In addition, the doctor under whose license our whole school functioned would be right down the hall.

The first thing you learn at a VA hospital is that you work for the government. This means that you have to fill out about nine hundred forms, which takes up most of any day. The upside is that you get paid real money, $12.50 an hour. This was going to be the most I had earned in several years. All right!

Joe and Dan took their role as preceptors seriously. They were still new enough at it to be very enthusiastic and I think they felt an obligation not to allow the program they'd come out of to turn out lunkheads.

They pimped me endlessly. It started when I got there and it would go on until I left at 5:00 p.m. That's another thing about the VA. You work full days, five days a week. No one takes an afternoon off to get in eighteen holes.

Some of my fellow students had not liked the pressure they felt during this rotation, especially being bombarded in front of patients with questions they couldn't answer. While I didn't relish it, I understood where my preceptors were coming from. After a while I started to see that I was getting better and thinking faster on my feet. They also gave nightly reading assignments. That sometimes interfered with cocktail hour.

As strict as these guys were, they also allowed me freedom in the hospital. They wanted me to know every inch of it and every department by the time that I left. They constantly encouraged me to go off and spend time with various doctors. One day I found my way down into the bowels of the place and walked into a dark room where the radiologist worked. He was an older guy who was probably past retirement age. I think he was still there, sitting in the ghostly light of the film viewers, because he had recently lost his wife; this helped keep his mind occupied. He seemed to like me personally. He would always say, "Stop in any time." I often did. We probably had more in common than if I was a twenty-something student. We talked politics and golf and the curve balls that life throws. He also taught me how to read an x-ray. They teach you that in the first year of school, but you don't really get it and are often lucky when you actually pick up an abnormality. He refined it for me. He said, "First you've got to know normal before you can spot abnormal." Next he taught me to approach every x-ray the same way and go over them each time in systematic fashion. You have to cover every inch. Just because you are looking for something in one area doesn't mean that you won't find things someplace else. He also pointed out different examples of why some shadows you might find on a lung x-ray were harmless and others were ominous. I'm still working on that part of my game. I always enjoyed sitting there in the glow with him. It was relaxing.

I did exams on about eleven patients a day. Most were elderly men with pretty much the same issues. Many of them had alcohol and tobacco related problems and most had a list of drugs they were on that looked like a small book. Invariably they'd tell you how proud they were to have served their country. Even though they felt they were owed this medical care, they almost always expressed appreciation for my services. They were all talkative and most were quite complementary of my skills. They were also interested in how someone who was their kids' age rather than their grandkids' age, was still a student. I told them I was a slow learner.

I had my only argument with a preceptor during this rotation. One day Dan said, "The charting you did on the last patient was lousy. Redo it." I was of the opinion that I had charted everything I could think of and that there was not much more to say on the matter. I voiced this to him in a fairly strong tone. He shot back with, "If you want to fuck up, do it on your own time. You're not going to do it on my watch." We went on in that vein for a while until I went and redid the notes. I had no hard feelings, but Dan was a little cool for a day or two. We got back on track, though. Guys have a way of working through stuff like that.

It was during this rotation that I was starting to feel that I didn't want to work in an office environment. I just didn't enjoy seeing a steady stream of patients who pretty much had the same issues. The fact that I was messed up in my personal life probably factored in there someplace too. Still I remember going to see my own doctor, Ron Witkin, for a physical. His practice is internal medicine. He was interested in how I was doing. I told him that I wasn't that into seeing a stream of eighty-year-old guys who all have heart disease, lung disease and enlarged prostates. He laughed. On the way out I said, "Maybe in a couple of months you ought to consider hiring a PA. He replied, "You're about my youngest patient. I think you just ruled yourself out of internal medicine a few minutes ago."

Mirno's office is in the same building as my doctor's. I stopped in to say hello. I told him how much I had loved surgery. He said, "If you liked that, you're probably going to like emergency medicine even more."

I don't recall many individual details in the internal medicine rotation. I saw a ton of patients, worked with a lot of different people in the hospital, and was made a better PA-in-training by two young PAs who thought it was important. I told them when I left, "I wasn't always thrilled with the method but you guys made me better. I appreciate that."

# Emergency Medicine

Most of our lectures in emergency medicine had been from a doctor who bore a striking resemblance to Santa Claus, with a thick white beard and flowing white hair that he wore on the longish side. He wasn't necessarily a jolly old elf but he was personable. His name was Alan Rogers. I had asked him at one time if he thought that I was too old for emergency medicine. I'd considered it to be a young person's domain. He was about my age. He said, "If you're healthy and have a strong work ethic, then age has nothing to do with it. The key is to get out of school and get a job with a great teacher. No one understands emergency medicine right off the bat. It takes a couple of years." I had filed that away but not given much more thought to emergency medicine.

I was now about to start my emergency rotation with the aforementioned Santa Claus. Even though this was June, he still had the regal bearing. He laid things out for me. "You don't have to wear your white coat if you don't want to, but I want you in a shirt and tie every day. You will work four shifts of twelve hours a day each week. You can work with any of the doctors that you like, but remember, I'm the one who'll be grading you." I think he had a better understanding than most preceptors that a student who was starting to get things could be a benefit to him rather than a hindrance. The hospital was in Claremont, NH, about a ninety-mile drive from my home. My shifts would be either from 8:00

a.m. to 8:00 p.m. or 12:00 to 12:00. I decided that a daily commute simply wasn't going to be feasible.

The only hotel I deemed to be up to my standards was situated across the street from the Sunapee ski area. Since this was the off season, their rate would only be $92.00 a night. Given that I was rapidly running out of money, that seemed exorbitant. I was in a race to see which would happen first: graduation or bankruptcy. I asked if they didn't have some kind of corporate rate for those of us working at Valley Regional Hospital. That got the rate reduced to $91.00 a night.

For my first day Dr. Rogers had me shadow him. He also made me pay for lunch, barbecue cooked on a smoker outside the hospital, and it was well worth every penny. I did a few minor procedures and then someone arrived with a pretty good cut on an arm. Dr. Rogers said, "I'll numb it and then you'll suture it." I was nervous. I wasn't yet confident in my sewing. I got it done but I was slow and my hands shook. The patient watched me like a hawk. I'd have to say that he didn't appear to have great faith in his medical provider. When we left the room Dr. Rogers said, "We need to work on that. Do you have a sewing board?" A sewing board has all sorts of foam pads and rubber tubing for you to sew together. I had one. He said, "Bring it in. I'll show you some technique for you to practice."

You sew by placing the needle into a needle holder with the thread trailing from it. The needle holder looks a little like a pair of needle-nose pliers with teeth in the grip and a ratchet in the handle. You only want to ratchet down enough to firmly hold the needle in place. If you ratchet down too tight you're guaranteed to have trouble releasing the needle after you come through the skin, resulting in your pulling the thread right through or losing the needle back into the skin while you're trying to get it to release. I had both of those things happen at various times while I struggled to loosen the needle. Secondly you want to have the needle enter the skin at a ninety degree angle so that when it comes out the other side it comes up smoothly and evenly spaced. Lastly you want to throw the knots that you make in the same way and same direction every time. Go back and reread the part about the trouble I had with knots at the ski area.

Part of sewing is purely functional. Part of it is artistic. When you are done everything should have an orderly and evenly spaced look to it. I was not there yet, not by a long shot. I already knew that I had to get better and was determined to. An emergency room is certainly the place to work on your sewing skills. Some days you deal with five or six bad cuts in a row.

The next day I worked with Dr. Joe Hagan. He'd been a doc in the navy for years; he still had that bearing about him. He could also be impatient, abrupt, and tough to stay with. He buzzed around like a mosquito. He was also a Philly guy with a Philly accent and a love for all things Philadelphia, especially sports, and he didn't care if it was schoolboy or pro. He was also opinionated on virtually any subject.

He backed these opinions with reasoning that sometimes bordered on brilliant. Trying to argue with him on most subjects was like getting into a gun fight only to discover that you'd loaded all your bullets into the gun you'd left at home.

For whatever reason, I loved this guy. To this day he is one of my favorite doctors. Maybe it's because he let me do a lot of stuff. Maybe it's because he occasionally cooked for me in the little kitchenette that was just off the department. Any patient that came in with nausea and vomiting on the days when he had his five alarm chili going out back was probably going to end up in intensive care rather than leave in an improved state.

The first day I worked with him a guy came in after having fallen off the roof of his sunroom. He had landed on a piece of sharp aluminum and had one of the nastiest, deepest cuts I'd seen to date, running from his knee halfway down his shin. Dr. Hagan said, "You can do this. Right?" I replied, "Sure." I knew that with him standing over my shoulder, I could get it done. He started to walk away. I asked, "Ahh, Doctor. Aren't you going to stay?" He replied, "Ger, the Red Sox game is tied." He went around the corner and disappeared into the doctors lounge. Thank God this patient was a tough cookie. I had to stick him about eleven times with a needle to get the whole area numbed. Either because of his thick skin or my technique, I bent two of the curved needles straight. It took me about half an hour, but I finally got about fifteen stitches into him and he never said a word except, "Thanks," when I was done. I went to get Dr. Hagan to sign off on what I had done. He took a quick look, said, "Looks great. Lets go make some chili." I gained huge confidence from that episode.

One morning a doctor who had his office across the street hobbled in. He had fallen down the stairs in his garage and as it turns out, fractured his ankle and ended up with a nasty cut in the palm of his hand. Dr. Rogers brought me into the room and said to him, "Frank, this is one of our students who's starting to get his technique down. I'm going to have him do your hand." The doctor said that'd be okay. Talk about shaky hands! This would be someone who'd be watching me with a very critical eye, indeed. I stuck the needle full of lidocaine into his palm and he grimaced. I said, "I'm sorry. I know this hurts." Through clenched teeth he said, "Keep going." I put four stitches in and was ready to go for a fifth when he said, "That's enough." I thought he hopped off the table a little quickly. I said, "Doctor, shouldn't you go home and get off that leg?" He mumbled, "Patients to see," and hobbled down the hall with his good hand on the wall.

One of the nurses had stayed in the room the whole time. She said to me, "I was rooting for you. I know how tough that must have been." I thanked her and replied, "I wish you had been holding me." She asked, "Didn't you feel my hand on your back?" I had been so focused in the moment that I noticed nothing but the hand that was attached to the doctor.

I started to realize during this rotation what a good nurse was and how invaluable a good nurse can be. We had a lot of good nurses in this emergency room. In my case they often saved me on those occasions when I hadn't a clue about something. I could be fumbling around about to prescribe for a patient and a nurse might say, "The last time you dealt with this, didn't you use Zithromax twice a day for seven days?" Oh yeah, of course I did. They also would do things like come into a room where I was getting ready to suture and say, "I was pretty sure that you wanted 4.0 thread and three cc's of lidocaine so that's what I've brought." Hey, you read my mind. They also typically have their own opinion about what's going on with a patient, and sometimes that can get you in trouble.

A patient came in. The nurse had been in to see him and told me, "I don't think there's anything wrong with this guy. I don't know why he's here." I went in to see the patient. He told me, "On Saturday I felt really tired and my stomach was bothering me. I'm starting to feel better now but I can't shake the tired feeling." I was thinking the problem was abdominal in nature. He also told me that he was a diabetic and that his father and two of his brothers had died from heart attacks when they were younger than he was. I wasn't thinking heart because he denied any chest pain or pain going into his neck or down his shoulder. Still, I ordered a test for troponin, among others. Troponin measures an enzyme that is released by damaged heart muscle and can be a pretty specific test for a heart attack. I did not order an EKG, where the electrodes get attached to your chest and you get a printout of the electrical activity of the heart. I went and told Dr. Horak what was going on and what I had ordered. First question: "Did you order an EKG?" I replied, "I don't think it's heart related so I didn't." He said, "You thought enough of it to order a troponin. Always order an EKG. They're cheap."

A little later, while he was reading the EKG I heard Dr. Horak say, "Buddy, you've had a heart attack." That's called learning from your mistakes.

Working an emergency room was my first real experience with drug seekers, a constant problem in every emergency department in the country. They can be quite sophisticated; they can also be very aggressive and demanding. As emergency department medical providers, we are all obligated to treat your pain. We are not obligated to always treat it with opioids. Let me state up front. I am in this business because I have a certain level of compassion for people who are suffering. Anyone in medicine has that attribute. The saying about "Who are you to judge someone else's pain" applies. If you have a condition which obviously causes pain, I am willing to give you enough pain killer to let you float above a field of daisies. The same applies if you look to be suffering and I don't yet know what's wrong with you.

On the other hand, there are certain patients who inspire a healthy level of skepticism. It's often the nurses who spot them. A nurse will tip you off with a, "See the person sitting by the door? He's been here five times in the past two weeks and the work-ups have always been negative for any findings, but he's usually left with a prescription for narcotics." As the provider, you hate to hear that sort of thing. I'm not your regular doctor or PA. I don't know your history. But now I'm suspicious. I go into the computer and pull up your record. Certain findings in previous visits don't jive. When I finally sit in a room and talk to you my thinking might change. Occasionally, just an unusual combination of odd circumstances have conspired to made you look bad. In those cases, I'll go ahead and treat you.

In other instances, the scenario goes like this: "I have a toothache." "Have you seen your dentist?" "I don't have one." I look in the patient's mouth, who may not have the best set of choppers in the world, but I don't see signs of the swelling and redness that typically go with a painful condition. I explain that to the patient. The patient replies, "Doc, you gotta help me. I'm in excruciating pain." I reply, "It's been found that a combination of extra-strength Tylenol and some Motrin works wonders for this. The patient replies, "Those drugs do nothing for me." You go through a list of other drugs, none of which have ever worked. Finally you ask, "What works?" "Percocet."

Percocet is a wonderful pain killer. For people who are in acute pain, it enables them to function on a day-to-day basis. If you are not really in pain (and, therefore, the drug doesn't attach to certain receptors) and you combine it with a couple of shots of gin, you'll feel capable of going to the moon without a rocket.

Another scenario involves the patient who comes in with awful pain of no known origin and brings a friend along with them. The friend is usually more aggressive than the patient in demanding that you treat this poor soul with narcotics. Call me cynical but that sets the red flags waving faster than anything. I might actually start to think, "Gee. If I write a script, the friend here's going to share in half of it."

Many of you reading this may be thinking to yourself, "Just where do you get off? You're a student, still wet behind the ears. The nerve of you." Well, you might be correct. At the same time, as I write this I am fifty-two years old. I read a lot. I'm also very inquisitive and have sat listening to the personal opinions of doctors on this subject, for hours on end. Also as this is being written I have been working in the field – but that's getting ahead of the story.

Excuse me while I get on my soapbox for a moment here. This is a huge problem. A lot of people go to emergency rooms just to get narcotics and often they do walk out with a prescription. Don't run to blame the doctors. They're trapped between the proverbial rock and a hard place. If they write scripts for too many narcotics, they can go to jail. If they hold back too often, someone will show up with a lawyer claiming that no one feels their pain. Hospital administrators don't like lawyers or TV crews, unless it's to talk about the incredible innovation that their hospital has just implemented.

Or how about this one. A patient comes in. One of the nurses goes in to see him. She comes out of the room and says, " I'm not buying this guy's story. I think it's bullshit." I go in to see him. The guy's grimacing with pain, says he'd been working under a buddy's car and the jack slipped. He'd been pinned but luckily was able to extricate himself. The story seems plausible. The patient looks to be really hurting. His right side doesn't seem to match up with his left side. My exam confirms that he's got a limited range of motion, loss of strength and reduced sensation on his right side. The x-rays don't show skeletal injury but I'm thinking there could be massive soft tissue damage. I go and tell Dr. Rogers what's going on. He sees the patient. Agreeing with my assessment, he cosigns my script for fifteen Percocet.

Two hours later we get a call from the local CVS. The pharmacist filled the prescription but he wants us to know that the same guy has come in during the past two weeks with other prescriptions – for a total of one hundred and twenty Percocet. I look at Dr Rogers. He looks at me. The nurse looks like the cat that swallowed the canary. We had most likely been had.

Our legislators in Washington need to be more aware of this problem. I bet that most of them have never spent much time in a hospital getting the real inside story. We don't need more laws. We need the laws that are already on the books clarified and enforced. I could write a lot more on this subject but I think that pretty much covers it...

All in all, I enjoyed this rotation a lot. The twelve-hour shifts could be wearing but I was learning with every patient I saw. I decided that emergency medicine was where I wanted to end up. I liked the adrenaline rush that came with not knowing what emergency might come through the door next, just like ski patrol. I liked the idea that you didn't have to do the typical follow-up that providers in primary care have to do. As somebody said, "You fix them, they get admitted or they die." That sounds a little cold and the person who said it didn't intend it to be. It was more of a comment on the realities of emergency medicine. I also liked the idea of not being on call. Your shifts might be long but when you were done, you were done.

Dr. Rogers gave me my review. He said, "Here's the deal. Personally, you're a pleasure to have around. You're good company. The nurses like you because you are willing to pitch in and do anything. However I'm not that impressed with your medical knowledge or skills. You're not as good as a medical student and you're not as good as a working PA. You still don't connect all the dots. You're average." It was the toughest evaluation that I'd been given so far.

There was a time when that evaluation would have really bothered me and in fact might have made me reconsider what I was doing. I was not deterred. I knew that I wanted emergency medicine. I wasn't a medical student although it would have been nice to have been told that I was as good as one. I also knew that I had time for improvement and that I would improve.

I marched on to my next rotation. I was going to a part of New Hampshire that many people don't know exists, an area called the Great North Woods.

# Family Medicine (Again)

Most people who come to New Hampshire finish their trek at the ocean, the Lakes Region or the White Mountains. This happens to be a state with some of the most beautiful scenery in the country. To get to where I was headed, you had to either go over the White Mountains or through them. Going through them meant passing through the Notches. 'Notch' is New Hampshire for mountain pass. We don't have mountains anywhere close to the size of those in the West, but we do have our own smaller and just as breathtaking version.

Coming down, or through, the other side of the White Mountains brings you into a sparsely populated  area of majestic woodlands, sprawling dairy farms, and undeveloped lakes and streams. The air smells different and it somehow seems quieter. Many of the people in this area make their living from the land, as farmers, loggers or both. One of my neighbors is a logger who spends a good part of each of his days in the woods. We were talking one day about how overrun our town was getting. He said, " If they put in one more traffic light I'm moving north." He was serious. The north he referred to was the area I'm describing.

These days, if you want to find the weathered, pipe-smoking fellow with the sharp accent that most folks imagine as the quintessential New Hampsherite, you'd have to come to the Great North Woods. The state motto is " Live Free or Die." Some parts of New Hampshire look on that scornfully. It is definitely trashed in some other states (a friend in Massachusetts refers to it as "Eat Shit and Die"). If you made fun of it up here, you'll hurt these folks' feelings. Some of them might also offer to whack you one in the mouth.

Driving the roads around here, I realized that my windshield had gotten really pitted by road salt. Sometimes the sun or oncoming headlights totally blinded me. I got a new windshield. People around here fear an encounter with a moose as much as people in desert areas fear an encounter with a rattlesnake. Driving into, or more likely under, a moose at sixty miles per hour can produce an equally dire outcome.

I was to spend the next five weeks in the Lancaster-Whitefield area with a doctor named John Ford. I had it in my mind from conversations with classmates that he'd be middle-aged, with about nine kids. I walked into his office and found a good-looking guy in his thirties with a goatee, wearing a short sleeved surgical top which revealed muscular arms. He looked like a light-weight boxer – there was a hint of the boxer's toughness about him. I thought, "Jesus, he's a kid." I introduced myself and he smiled warmly, which brought out the deep crows feet around his eyes. He said, "Hi," in a soft voice.

This would be my second family practice rotation. He said, "Before you get all comfortable we have to run up to the hospital. We're going to deliver a baby." I followed him out and got into his car. As we made the nine-mile drive from his office to the hospital, he explained the case. We wouldn't actually be doing the delivery. It was going to be by caesarean section and we would take responsibility for the baby once the obstetrician had done the surgery. The mother had several children under the age of five and had never seen a doctor during the pregnancy. There would probably be complications.

We drove up and down mountains with panoramic views of other mountains and towns nestled in valleys. At one point, Dr. Ford said, "That's Vermont over there." We passed a deer standing in the middle of an open field and some wild turkeys milling around on the side of the road. He didn't seem to notice them. We came down a steep hill into the middle of Lancaster, which had the look of the classic New England town from the movies, all tree-lined and brick. It even had an old fashioned drug store that didn't have one of the national chain names across the top of it. We went up the road and passed signs for the hospital and pulled into the parking lot of a small but new- looking facility. He parked in a space with a sign that read, "Reserved for emergency room physician."

We walked into the building through a blast of air conditioning and ran up a flight of stairs. This place didn't have the hustle and bustle I was used to in other hospitals – it was more like the atmosphere in the main room of a bed and breakfast. We went around a corner and through a pair of big fire doors with signs that read, "Authorized personnel only." A nurse in surgical scrubs said, "Hi, John. They're just getting started." We went into the locker room, got undressed, and started putting on the garb that by now felt quite comfortable to me. I felt foolish in my Gucci street shoes. Dr. Ford had on beat up old Topsiders. We didn't bother with shoe covers. We scrubbed up and then backed into the operating room.

The mother was lying on the table, all draped, talking to the obstetrician. She'd been given a spinal anesthetic so she was asleep from her chest down. The rest of her was quite awake. She looked weathered, but otherwise pretty young.

Not wasting any time, the ob made a long incision across her lower abdomen. The doctor who was assisting him used a couple of retractors to stretch the layers of skin apart, then the ob went in after the baby. It appeared he was having to struggle to get it out. At one point he just about had it by the feet and bottom but it slid back in. The baby was overdue and quite large. Finally the baby popped out and was immediately handed to us. While the docs at the table worked on closing the mother's abdomen, we set to getting this little fellow started in the world. He didn't move at all and was blue – he wasn't breathing. Dr. Ford told me to suction out his mouth. I did this, but again there was no reaction from the baby. Dr. Ford stuck his finger into the little mouth and fished around. To this point, the little guy still hadn't uttered a peep. Dr. Ford said, "I'm going to have to intubate." A respiratory therapist joined us with a kit that contained what looked like miniature scale versions of the equipment I had seen used so often on adults. Dr. Ford got a breathing tube into the baby faster than I'd ever seen it done. The respiratory therapist started squeezing on the little plastic bag that was attached to the even smaller tube in the baby's mouth. The mood was just this side of relaxed, but grim and determined. I was already rooting for this little guy who hadn't existed five minutes ago.

The baby sort of yawned around the tube but still didn't cry or move. I kept repeating to myself, "Please don't die." His color got a little better but his vital signs weren't good. It was decided to take him from his mother and down to the nursery. The team moved as one as we wheeled him in a little incubator out of the operating room and down the hall. The nursery, a warm and softly lit room, had all sorts of equipment and monitoring devices in it. We kept working and I took over the rhythmic squeezing of the breathing bag. His vital signs would start to approach normal but then fall back. I don't think that his blood pressure or oxygen saturation ever got close to where they needed to be.

It was decided that the little guy would have to be transferred to neonatal intensive care at Dartmouth Hitchcock. A call was placed for the helicopter. Dr. Ford continued to work on the baby. Even though things weren't right, we still had basic issues to address. He talked me through the exam that's done on all newborns to determine if all the parts are present and in working order. He also said, "I'm pretty sure this baby has Downs syndrome." After a while the helicopter team marched in wearing their forest green flight suits and engineer boots. I don't care who you are. You put on one of those uniforms and you exude confidence and coolness. I made a mental note to ask Dr. Ford if I could wear one back at his office.

The flight team would now take responsibility for our little patient. Dr. Ford started signing documents and giving them his report at the same time. A nurse came in and told him that the father wanted to talk to him. We went out into the hall. A young man stood against the wall holding two toddlers by their hands. He asked, "Is there something wrong with my baby?" Dr. Ford explained that there were some issues that required more than we could offer, so the baby was being airlifted to another hospital. The father said, "Okay. I've got to get these kids fed. I'll be at McDonalds." He walked out. The flight team hurried by, pushing our little guy in an incubator. We didn't say anything to them. He was no longer our patient. We went over to a large picture window and stared down into the parking lot where an orange chopper sat with the blades kicking up a dust storm. After a minute, the flight crew appeared as they wheeled their special cargo across the parking lot. We watched as they loaded him in and then took what seemed to be forever to take off. Dr. Ford stood with his hands folded across his chest. He never moved. As the helicopter took off he said, "Imagine only being on this earth for one hour and already you don't have a chance in hell." He shook his head.

All doctors work hard, but John Ford worked more hours in more places than any of the preceptors I spent the year with. The typical day started at the hospital around 6:30. We did rounds on any of his patients who were there. I did most of the exams and most of the charting. He'd then make the perfunctory visit in each room and then often make me rewrite what I had charted. We'd then head to his office for what was typically a nine to five day of patient visits. In between we'd make two or three trips back to the hospital to admit patients or because some emergency had cropped up with a patient who was already there. We also regularly made the drive to the local nursing home where he had a number of patients. On top of that, he worked a twenty-four hour shift in the emergency room once a month.

As we got to be more familiar with each other, we both started to fill in the blank spaces about ourselves. We had some great talks, almost always on the run. He had grown up hard, had gotten married young and was now going through a divorce. There weren't nine kids. There was one: a teenage son. He revered his kid.

He was the most unique doc that I got to spend time with. John Ford, the doctor, would fit the bill of the old-time doc you might find in a John Ford, the director, movie. He was the doc who often brought someone into the world and pulled the sheet over an older face after a last torturous breath. He's a hunter, and an avid one at that. During this period of time he was also an enthusiastic consumer of chewed tobacco products, the production of which he would spit into styrofoam cups. I could often follow him around the hospital by following a trail of such cups, each with what appeared to be that last gulp of morning coffee. More than once I had to jump towards a nurse and say, "That's not your coffee!" No one was bothered by any of this. Imagine that being the attitude at Massachusetts General Hospital!

Apparently my initial take on John Ford looking like a boxer wasn't far off. He told me he'd done some boxing. He also told me there was a time in his life when he'd really enjoyed the occasional old-fashioned barroom brawl, with folks flying over tables and whatnot. I asked if he still engaged in that sort of thing. He replied, "Nah. Bad for business."

## Family Medicine (Again) Becomes Women's Health

About a week into this rotation I got a call from the school. They said, "Listen. We're having a problem getting men placed into women's health rotations, and you're no exception. See if Dr. Ford is willing to change this from family practice to women's health." I felt like an ass having to go and have this conversation. He laughed. He said, "Nothing will change. You're still going to spend most of your time with elderly men who have congestive heart failure. I'll try to make sure that you do an exam on every woman who walks through the door."

This rotation confirmed that I wanted to work in a hospital environment. I looked forward to the morning rounds and I really enjoyed the occasional twenty-four hours of emergency room duty. The office time had become a bit tedious. One day I told Dr. Ford, "I'm starting to feel a little burned out." He laughed, somewhat surprised, and said, "You can't be burned out. You're just a student." I tried to explain to him that it had been a long time since I'd had a vacation and also that I was narrowing down the career paths I saw for myself in medicine. I still had tons to learn. I didn't want him to think that I now viewed myself as any kind of hotshot student.

If I was a rough jewel in need of finishing, Dr. Ford was the jeweler to start chipping off large chunks of rough edges. Among several of my bad habits, one really stood out – it had already been pointed out by the nursing advisor who had not been my biggest fan: I tended to jump to conclusions. Often, when I didn't know what I was dealing with and thus didn't have a clue as to what I was talking about, I would, undeterred, talk myself into a certain position and, once it started sounding good to me, I'd set to selling my preceptor on it. I was sufficiently aware of this to, at times, ask myself, "Okay. Do you know what you're doing or are you just trying to sell your way through all of this?"

Dr. Ford put an end to this. One day I was rambling my way down a country road of thought that was really starting to make sense to me. Dr. Ford gave me a look, the visual equivalent of being shaken by the shoulders, and yelled, "Stop selling me! You're not in the toy business anymore. Either you know it or you don't. If you don't know it, then go read up on it before you present it to me." He was right. I went and did some reading and then went back and started selling him on why I was right and the book was wrong. He closed his eyes and held the bridge of his nose between his thumb and forefinger.

Under his tutelage I started to make the transition from student to someone who made decisions on his own and then started to formulate a plan. This is a major transition point for any student learning his craft. Dr. Ford would occasionally say, "I'm not always going to be around for you. You know that the time is coming when you are going to be doing this for real and will have to live with your decisions." That thought was way too scary to contemplate.

He challenged me constantly. Not so much pimping, but true challenges on diagnoses and plans to improve patient outcomes. It was painful, but my improvement started coming, an inch at a time.

From a medical standpoint, Dr. Ford may have been the smartest doctor that I got to spend time with. I was at a point where I was starting to ask some pretty sophisticated questions. Some of them required involved formulas to answer. He never hesitated once before giving me a reply and often would sit down and do a complicated schematic of a formula on a napkin. I still have those.

One day he said, "Your first patient today is a retired doctor who's here for a physical. This will be a good experience for you." Maybe he thought so. I figured this was going to be an opportunity to be exposed for all that I didn't know. I walked into the examining room to find a gentleman in his seventies sitting there wearing brightly colored suspenders. I introduced myself as a student. He said, "Please don't use big words. You students often confuse me with terminology." He flashed a wry grin. I asked him the standard questions that all patients are asked as part of a health history. Since he was a doctor I almost passed over the one about, "Do you smoke?" I asked it in an almost 'aw shucks' manner. His reply was, "Yup." I looked up in surprise. He shrugged his shoulders. I asked him how much he smoked. He said, "A pack a day for, oh, I dunno, about fifty-five years." I asked, "Do I need to talk to you about smoking?" He replied, "Maybe. Can you teach me anything about it?" That wry smile again. I said, "Well, ultimately it is probably going to be the thing that kills you." He shot back with, "Well, there's news!" I was reminded of a question I had asked the doctor with the Prussian accent who had lectured us about lung function. I had asked, "Doctor, I know that we're supposed to counsel all patients on smoking cessation. However, if you've got someone who's smoked heavily for their whole life, will it make much of a difference?" He thought for a moment and replied, "No. The patient is kaput!"

One Friday as I was getting ready to leave and head back to the Lakes Region, Dr. Ford said, "I know that you old guys need your rest but if you feel like doing some emergency room time, I'm on this weekend." Excited, I said, "Definitely." He said, "See you Sunday morning at 8:00." On Sunday I left home at about 6:00 to make the drive back to the hospital. I grabbed some breakfast in the cafeteria and joined Dr. Ford in the E.D. We were busy right from the start. I did a lot of suturing and a number of procedures. I also correctly diagnosed a patient with a pulmonary embolism. Before I knew it, midnight had come and gone. At about 2:00 a.m. it was very quiet and Dr. Ford said, "I'm going to get some sleep. Why don't you go upstairs to the residents' room and do the same." He went off to the doctors' room which was just off of the E.D. and shut the door. I went up the stairs to the residents' room, only to find the door closed and locked. Damn. Someone had beaten me to it. I went back down to the E.D. and asked one of the nurses what she thought I should do. She said, "Why don't you try the nursery. They usually have a bed." I went back up the stairs to the obstetrics lounge and talked to a nurse. She said, "We've had several women come in since yesterday afternoon. There aren't any beds." Double damn. I looked down the hall to what appeared to be an empty room. I asked, "What about down there?" She said, "That's a birthing bed." I replied, "That'll do." She said, "If you say so." We walked down to the room and she got me a pillow. As she was walking out she asked, "Are you sure?" I said, "Yeah. No problem."

I had never been on a birthing bed. This is a piece of equipment designed to provide plenty of support for a woman in labor. I don't think the idea that someone might actually try to sleep on one had ever been factored in. It was like laying on a slab of warm concrete. After about an hour of tossing and turning I found some semblance of comfort and dozed off fitfully. I don't think I ever really conked out. I was afraid that if I started snoring, I'd wake up all the expectant mothers. After about two hours of this I got up and staggered around until I found the shower. I decided the hell with a shower and headed down to the emergency department. All was quiet and there was no sign of Dr. Ford. I decided to start rounds a little early. I did exams on four very grumpy patients and charted the medication orders and procedures that needed to be done. I headed back down to the E.D. Still no sign of Dr. Ford. I went and grabbed some breakfast and sat trying to wake up. At about ten to eight I went back and knocked on his door. I heard some rustling. After a few minutes he came out looking bleary-eyed, stretching like an old cat. He asked, "How'd you sleep?" I grunted a reply. We went back to the medical floor so he could review what I had done. Once he decided that everything was in order, we walked out into the cool, sunny morning and headed to his office. We would now work a nine to five shift there.

At about 2:30, I was really dragging but trying not to show it. At one point he walked into his office and said, "Man, I'm really tired. How are you feeling?" I replied, "I feel great." He said, "I don't know how you do it." He walked out. I immediately put my head down on his desk, trying not to make too much noise when it landed. I was out on the spot.

As I look back, some of the best times that I had were working those all-night shifts with Dr. Ford. Often our main pursuit would be in finding something to eat in the middle of the night. The hospital would be deathly quiet as we went slinking around the halls like a couple of mice. These late night snacks – apple juice, peanut butter on crackers and a vanilla Dixie Cup – reminded me of sleepovers and raiding the refrigerator when you are seven.

I got along great with the staff in his office. They seemed to love having students around and thought we were all cute, even us fifty-one-year-olds. I tend to be reserved around people until I get to know them. Because of this and because I don't think they yet got my sense of humor, they decided that I was shy.

Since this was now my women's health rotation, I had to do a number of pelvic exams. As I write this, I've done enough of them that it's become pretty much just another procedure. At that time, I really would have preferred not to do any. The staff knew that and I think that added to the impression of shyness. One day I was about to go into a room to perform one and the medical assistant, Kim, asked, "Are you going in?" She meant it as "in" the room. I thought she meant it as "in" like in as part of the exam. I sighed and resignedly said, "Yes. I'm going in." It only took a second before we realized that we had both meant something very different. From then on the rallying cry was, "So, Gerry, are you going in?"

The rotation was wrapping up and I had really gotten to like the area and the medical staff at the office and the hospital. I was thinking that it would be a great place to work even though the commute would be a challenge. Dr. Ford hooked me up with Dr. Johnson, who ran the emergency department. I had done some time with him on Dr. Ford's few days off. He told me that because it was such a small emergency department, they didn't really have a need for a PA However, he said he'd make some calls to friends in other departments. I felt like that was progress.

# Family Health (Again), Again

I got ready for my next rotation, which would be family health again. It was now late August. I would still be in northern New Hampshire, but where I had just been on the western border near Vermont, I'd now be on the eastern border near Maine. I would spend all of my time in the Berlin/Gorham area. Gorham is a major-league ski town. The peaks of the White Mountains caromed skyward across the street from the hotel where I would be staying. Eight miles up the road was Berlin, a tough, old mill town. The Androscoggin river, complete with rapids and small waterfalls, runs through town. Beside it sits a large paper mill which has experienced several changes of ownership. With each change, the town and the mill seemed to struggle a little bit harder. On a good day, the area around the mill smelled. On a bad day it really smelled. People liked to refer to it as the smell of money. I once knew a guy who pumped out septic tanks who said the same thing. As so often happens in these environments, people who've lived with it for a long time don't even notice the odor. I wouldn't live with it that long.

Nestled on a rise above the mill and just south of a maximum security prison is Androscoggin Valley Hospital. Most days the prevailing wind blew away from the hospital. On my first day there, I met Grant Niskanen, M.D., at 8:00 a.m. in the hospital cafeteria. Another small hospital that looked brand new, it appeared to be a little busier than the one I'd just left. Dr. Niskanen was tall and gangly, with a great tan, though he didn't look particularly athletic. Again, appearances can be deceiving. The tan came from golf. I was told by a doctor who often played with him that when he was on his game he was unbeatable. He regularly hit drives as long as any pro's. I was also told that when he was not on his game, the mild mannered doctor could turn into a bear.

After I got to know him, I found the bear part hard to imagine. He was the easiest-going doctor I would work with all that year. His attitude was that you are only a student once. When you start working for real, you basically sacrifice your time and life to medicine. When he worked, it was nonstop. When he played, it seemed to be with the same ethic. He rarely ate lunch – he was usually at the golf course hitting a bucket of balls. He told me that although he enjoyed downhill skiing, he preferred cross country. He didn't ski at a leisurely pace, either. He went out every time with the idea of besting his own record. He said that he could go uphill faster than he could come down the other side, and uphill around these parts should not be underestimated. He also told me that he had run track at the University of Maryland. One of his teammates was Renaldo Nehemiah, who'd gone on to success as an Olympic hurdler. He had also been one of the first track men drafted into pro football. The problem seemed to be that he outran most passes thrown to him.

The routine with Dr. Niskanen was one that was now becoming, well, routine. We'd meet at the hospital for rounds. Then it was off to the office for a full day.

One or two days a week were spent completely at the hospital, days when he would do circumcisions and colonoscopies. They were the best days. First off, I was in my favorite environment. Secondly we were usually done by 1:30 and, as he rushed off to the golf course, I'd get to drive home through one of the most spectacular mountain passes in the east. On one side of the road was the Wildcat ski area. On the other was Mount Washington, which rose up from the road so quickly and steeply that I couldn't see the top even by leaning way into the windshield. I would often pull into the Wildcat parking lot just to stare for a while. This being toward the end of the summer, it was perfectly still and quiet. Looking up at the summit, I could often see a wisp of clouds that seemed to simply materialize there. It meant the jet stream was acting up and that conditions up there were probably just a bit more chaotic than down in the quiet parking lot. I also noticed that some of the leaves were starting to show hints of changing color. Winter does indeed come early to these parts.

In terms of medical philosophy, Dr. Niskanen was a minimalist. That's to say, he believed that the human body was capable of great things – including curing itself of many issues if given enough time and rest. He wasn't keen on prescribing $100 medication if an aspirin could produce the same outcome. Of course he did it from time to time, but he was not a doctor who spent all day reaching for his prescription pad. I liked his thinking enough that I decided that I'd emulate his philosophy. The difference was that he knew what he was doing and I still pretty much didn't. I just filed the observation away for future reference.

He liked to pimp and he'd pepper me with questions first thing in the morning. Trust me, that wakes you up real quick. After a while I found that incorporating his philosophy into my answers made for some modest successes. If I didn't know something I would answer, "That drug makes no difference or, the procedure doesn't need to be done." That got me several "Attaboy's."

Sometimes I'd say something to him or ask a question which resulted in a sharply delivered, "What?" I wondered what I might have said wrong. Eventually I found out that he was hard of hearing in one ear. Since I was a little concerned about my own hearing and the idea that I might miss an important sound in my stethoscope, I asked him about it. He replied that one of the best cardiologists he'd ever known was almost stone deaf. He relied on what he saw and felt and read from tests. That made me feel a little better.
One day, after having seen him do a number of circumcisions, I said, "Doc, why don't you take a breather. I'll do the next one." I was kidding. He replied, "Jesus, the nurses would kill me if I ever let a student do one. They're very protective of those little pee-pees."

By his estimation he had done close to a thousand colonoscopies. If you've never had one, I can tell you it's no big deal, and that's also from personal experience.

You are consciously sedated with Ativan and Versed. Even if you wake up during the procedure and start to squirm, you won't remember it when it's over. The key to a successful procedure – your preparation the night before has left you with a sparklingly clean colon. This is accomplished by drinking a couple of liters of what amounts to Drano for humans. It doesn't taste great but it's not awful. You'll spend a couple of hours in the bathroom with a mild but persistent case of diarrhea, guaranteed.

The next day you come into the hospital and are brought to the operating area. An I.V. is started and you get a steady amount of drugs until you just don't care about much of anything. You're then wheeled into an operating room for the procedure, which is not, by its very nature, considered a sterile procedure, nor is the staff performing it concerned about sterile fields. The scope, a thin black tube calibrated with measurement, has a control box on the end of it that doesn't differ much from a video game joy stick. This allows the doctor to turn the scope in different directions, insert air, inject water, and suck air and water out. It also contains a T.V. camera and a cutting apparatus for removing bits of tissue and small polyps. Obviously, it requires a certain amount of dexterity on the part of the operator. As mundane, or more likely gross, as you might find the subject, no two colons are alike and there's always the potential of perforating the intestine. Then you have a medical emergency.

As sick as this may sound to you, I always got a kick out of watching Dr. Niskanen do this procedure. He'd insert the scope with one gloved hand while rapidly cranking away on the joy stick with the other, all of this while never looking at the patient. Instead, he was focused on the T.V. screen above his head, giving us real-time pictures of the patient's colon. He transformed before our eyes from a skilled doctor into nine-year-old boy playing a complicated video game. His hands were a flurry of activity, his face a mask of concentration. His tongue usually protruded from between his teeth. Once, after the remnants of some bowel content had temporarily clouded the camera, he exclaimed, "Oh, no. We've been attacked by a death star!"

I asked him if I could do one, and this time I wasn't kidding. He said, "No." He added, "You probably could get it done on some level, but as you know there's potential for huge complications. Also you have to have done enough of them to know what's normal and what needs to be biopsied. I wouldn't have the same feel standing here guiding you through it, and there's too much at stake. Besides, as it stands today, PAs aren't authorized to do them, so you don't need to learn." Probably just as well. I stink at video games.

The people that I saw back at Dr. Niskanen's office were pretty much out of the same mold. This will be a generalization, but it works. Most of them were of French-Canadian heritage. They were tough, physical people, not that far removed from their ancestors who carved out a life in a difficult environment, and they were, for the most part, extremely street-smart. Most didn't go to the doctor because they had nothing else to do. More likely, they were there because something was really wrong or the doctor had called and said, "Since you haven't had a physical in twelve years, maybe it's time?" Invariably they were appreciative of my services and were open to suggestions about health improvement as long as the suggestions in question weren't judgmental. I liked these people a lot.

Where Dr. Ford hacked away at the rough stone that was me, Dr. Niskanen started to polish it. Other students had found their time with him very demanding. I found it effortless. He was the first doc to really take time with me on my charting. He was concerned about it from a history and legal standpoint, but even more so from a get-paid standpoint. Insurance companies pay out on what is charted. If you forget to dot an i or cross a t, they may very well deduct twenty bucks from what they pay out. As much as we all are in this profession for the good of mankind, we have to eat. He told me not to forget that. "A poor medical provider can be a desperate medical provider."

This rotation was almost over. I had yet to hear from the school as to where I was going next. I had completed every rotation except for pediatrics and my elective, which I knew was going to be emergency medicine. One night I was talking to Rick Miga, who'd been my college roommate for a couple of years. At one time we'd been extremely close, "as thick as thieves," as the movie *Shawshank Redemption* called it. We had drifted apart a bit but could still talk a couple of times a year and pick up right where we'd left off. I was telling him that I felt the school wasn't getting it done for me just when I needed to call on them the most. He said, "Hell, my brother Danny's a pediatrician in Denver. I'm sure he'd take you on."

Danny Miga was four years old the last time I'd see him. He used to run around the living room in nothing more than his Batman underwear, of which he seemed quite proud. The Dr. Miga that I talked to on the phone sounded a little more mature; if he was wearing Batman underwear, I was pretty sure it was well hidden under several layers of clothing. He told me that he vaguely remembered me throwing him down the cellar stairs and would like to return the favor as a preceptor. I could live with him and his family. I was excited. I called my school. They said they'd prefer that I stay on this side of the Mississippi, so they could more closely monitor my progress. Rats. I hadn't been to Denver in several years and was kind of getting in the mindset to go. At the same time, my money was going out in hemorrhagic quantities, so this wasn't the worst news in the world. They asked me if I had any other ideas. I said, "Well, when I was with Dr. Ford I did more exams on little kids than I did on women. Maybe I can go back there." They said that they'd call him.

I called Dr. Miga back and thanked him but told him I wouldn't be coming west. He sounded disappointed. I have a feeling that his wife was relieved.

Christy and I had begun inching back towards each other. The occasional phone call with its "How are things?" had turned into more serious conversations. We realized that we couldn't spend the rest of our lives acting like two love-drunk teenagers. We also acknowledged that on some level we were addicted to each other. Attempts at finding replacements for each other just didn't feel right. We decided that, as two strong-willed people trying to co-exist, we would always have our ups and downs – but that it was worth another try. Here we went again.

# Pediatrics

Dr. Ford was willing to take back a student he'd already had. I walked into his office on a Monday morning with a big smile on my face. He said, "I wish they'd told me who the student was when I still had a chance to say no!" His expression, however, said he was happy to see me. I know that I drove him nuts at times but I was pretty sure that he liked having me around.

He said, "You already know the routine. You'll see anybody and everybody who comes through this office. I'll try to make sure that you do lots of physicals on kids and see anything of particular interest." He was right. I already knew the routine. He also said that, whereas my last time with him had entailed tons of hours, this rotation was going to be somewhat fragmented. After all, it was hunting season; he'd be spending a good many of his vacation hours in the woods. This presented a bit of a problem. The school mandated that you had to be with your preceptor for just about every hour that he worked and that you had to have a minimum of one hundred and sixty hours over the course of the rotation. The last time I had been with Dr. Ford, we'd totaled over two hundred and twenty hours together. His schedule for the next five weeks looked like it would come down to about one hundred and forty hours. He said, "No problem. You can fill in the rest by going up to the emergency department and working with Dr. Johnson. He seems to tolerate you." That worked.

When you've spent most of your time listening to the sick lungs and hearts of chronically ill older folks, it is a little bit startling to suddenly hear and feel the bodies of vibrantly healthy patients, which for the most part is what I found in pediatrics. Even when kids are sick – and kids can go down the drain real fast – they still had that fresh-from-the-factory look and feel to them. Kids usually tell you right away if they're sick or not. Their color is off. They lie still in their parents arms and aren't very approachable. They don't display the normal inquisitiveness that healthy kids show you. Even at this stage I could walk into a room and immediately tell if I was dealing with a problem or just an overly concerned parent. Usually, after I'd assured the parents that this probably wasn't a big deal, and then gotten Dr. Ford to reinforce what I was saying, they'd turn sheepish and start apologizing for coming in. This would require several more minutes reassuring them that they'd done the right thing. A rule of thumb seems to be in play here: the number of trips to the doctor goes down proportionally with the number of kids in the family. With enough practice, most moms become pretty good pediatricians.

I saw a lot of kids having kids, moms who were eighteen or younger. Sometimes a young father would come along; many of them looked like they hadn't needed to shave yet. Dr. Ford often found himself teaching the most basic concepts, like understanding that the baby was fussy because it was hungry. More than once, I observed him teaching these youngsters how to feed and when to feed.

Initially, I was impressed that these kids cared enough to keep their babies and were trying to make a home for them. After giving it some thought, though, and factoring in some of my own life experiences, I found my viewpoint changing a bit. I'd think, "Jeez, just when you're starting to grow up and should be out having fun with your friends, you're going to be home most nights with one or more cranky, sniffling kids." I rank the old saying, "if you're old enough to make a baby, you're old enough to take care of it," right up there with a lot of other less than 100% reliable folk wisdom. Often grandmas in their forties would be part of the picture, rarely looking exactly thrilled. They knew all too well the role that lay ahead for them, in an area of responsibility they'd figured was behind them.

The end of October was approaching. In the North Country, fall foliage season peaks several weeks earlier than further south. There were still patches of beautiful color lighting up the woods and mountains, but for the most part, it looked more and more like what the more southerly portions of New England thought of as the look of Thanksgiving. Halloween had yet to arrive; farmhouses still had their corn stalks and stacks of pumpkins scattered about. The nights were crisp with frost and the air had that earthy, mulch-laden smell of New England at this time of year. From a weather standpoint, nature was confused: the transition from late summer and early fall into winter is never a smooth one in these parts. One day you'd be treated to bright sunlight and big puffy clouds. The next could be raw and windswept with rain. The winds of November that Gordon Lightfoot wrote about aren't exclusive to Lake Superior. Just before Halloween that year, most of New Hampshire got an early Nor'easter, with pouring cold rain. I was driving back up from the Lakes Region at the tail end of this storm. As I climbed in elevation, winter began to show its face; snow and sleet started to clog my windshield wipers. A few miles further and I was full into mid-winter. Drifts of snow were piled on the side of the road where plows had pushed them. The pumpkins on the front steps of houses wore eight-inch caps of the stuff. As I descended into the valley, fall returned with the remnants of green lawns and brightly colored leaves scattered around the yards. In my rear view mirror I could see the snow capped summits of the White Mountains when they peeked through the clouds. Two different seasons in the span of one set of eyes – how cool.

Dr. Ford spent most of this time sneezing and blowing his nose from having spent too many hours sitting in the woods with cold rain running down the back of his neck. Apparently he wasn't bothered by this; he kept going back. He said that the hunting wasn't all that good this year. A warm fall had produced an abundance of nuts and berries, so most of the deer and bear were staying way deep in the woods. He wasn't even bothered, or injured, when his friend shot him, Dick Cheney style, in the backside with birdshot. He told me that it happens pretty regularly; usually no harm is done. One day we were sitting in his office having one of our occasional yacks about non-medical stuff. I told him that I myself could never hunt but that I felt that hunters provided a valuable service to the ecosystem; with predators gone, the herds had to be thinned somehow. The thought or sight of starving deer staggering around or being brought down by roaming dogs who'd lost their own instinctual sharpness for doing this, made me sick. He leaned way back in his chair with his fingers locked behind his head. He said, "If you really think about it, any pursuit we engage in from the time we're born is just filling time until we die." It took several hours for my normal, optimistic equilibrium to return.

Dr. Ford kept hunting and I moved on to my final rotation. I realized that this year was all about spending time with a number of different medical providers, but I couldn't help but feel let down by the fact that I would never see some of them again. You spend enough time with some people and it becomes personal. For them, it's an endless line of students they never refuse, one pretty much the same as the next.

## Elective Rotation: Emergency Medicine (Again)

I was now in the home stretch. No checkered flags were being waved, but there was no way I wasn't going to graduate now. After two days of vacation I walked into Valley Regional Hospital again. Nothing had changed. The hours were the same but the days were much shorter. I got there at daybreak and I left in darkness. There was a new doc, last name of Mills, who I worked with the first few days of the rotation. He was soft spoken and smiled softly, too, but often. He was completely nonjudgmental of my skills and knowledge. He only commented on things if I asked him a question or needed an explanation of something. I thought, "Well, maybe that's just his personality." The other thought I had was that since I was just about done with school, he assumed that I would pretty much know what I was doing. It occurred to me that before too long, I'd be doing this for a living. I would then be a for-real PA. Nobody would be looking over my shoulder all day. Doctors would not tolerate me running to them every two minutes with questions, when I should know the answers. That was disconcerting.

I worked with my true preceptor, Dr. Rogers, for the next few days. At the end of the first day he said, "Your knowledge and skills have come a long way." That meant a lot to me. I had purposely asked to come back to this site for my final rotation. Dr. Rogers had been my toughest critic during the year and I knew he wouldn't pull any punches with me now.

He and I talked about how the baseball season had ended up. Not professional baseball – his baseball. He played in an over-forty league that included some ex-major leaguers. The first day that I had worked with him back in June, he had tried to sign me up. He said, "You look like a pitcher." I had in fact been one. He said, "We need pitching help." I told him that because of too many years spent in weight rooms, I was pretty sure I could no longer reach home plate, let alone "bring it" with the old fastball. I like to think that my refusal was the reason he'd been such a tough grader.

Maybe because the weather was getting cold, or maybe it was because of that phase of the moon, we started to get a lot of "frequent flyers," those folks known by everyone because they grace the emergency department with such regular visits. Some of them are the drug seekers I've already mentioned. Some were there for what is referred to as 'secondary gain' – the satisfaction and reassurance they get from the attention, even when that attention involves needles and invasive procedures. Sometimes the attention is brusque and rude, but they still come back. Who knows – maybe they're just lonesome.

Unfortunately an emergency department is not a social club. Sometimes it is super busy, with everyone trying to juggle more really sick people than they can handle. The doctors and nurses are tired and on edge; tempers grow short. In the middle of all of this an ambulance crew calls in to let you know they're on their way with patient so-and-so, a name that produces audible groans and the occasional swear word. Many of these folks always arrive by ambulance, a $500 taxi ride that ultimately gets paid for by John Q. Public, and is now an ambulance that's tied up for an hour on what is most likely a non-medical issue. How would you feel if one of your loved ones keeled over at the kitchen table and you were told that an ambulance would be dispatched "when available?"

The patient is brought in and, since he came by ambulance, he takes precedence over the guy who's been sitting patiently in the waiting room for an hour with blood soaking through his bath towel after that little oops he made with his circular saw.

The patient who just came in by ambulance is wheeled into a room. You ask him what's going on. You get a vague and general complaint that you've heard from him ten times before, but it usually includes a detail or two that could point to something that might be potentially serious. So you order an EKG and maybe a CT scan, and you do lots of blood workups. The meter is running the entire time, of course. Counting the ambulance ride, you're probably already looking at a bill for two grand. Typically, all of your findings will come back normal, or at least unchanged from previous workups, but you have to do all of this because, God forbid, the one time you don't take it seriously and there is really something going on, the lawyers will end up fighting for parking spaces in front of the hospital.

And this is just one scenario. Every hospital in America regularly deals with ten to twenty patients who fit this profile, showing up on a regular basis. Do the math, and you'll no longer need to wonder why the cost of your medical care is so high.

After dealing with one such patient one morning, I said to Dr. Hagan, "I know that, as a student, it's wrong for me to feel as cynical as I do right now." He lectured me, "Ger, you can't be cynical in this business. That patient has some issues and is lonely, and we're probably the only family she has. Be compassionate." I felt ashamed.

Five minutes later, however, I passed her room and heard the doctor lecturing this same patient. His face grew red as he said, "This crap has got to stop. From now on if you want to come running in here, please, take a cab."

Later I asked him why we couldn't just charge every patient that came in, just some nominal amount even, say, ten dollars. The reply was, "That'd probably actually be enough to make this a profitable emergency room, except for one little problem: we'd lose our federal funding." An emergency room is the last stop for some people, where all will get treated whether they can pay or not. Most emergency rooms I'd worked in had signs posted to that affect.

Once again, I stayed most nights at the hotel across the street from Mount Sunapee. This being late November, the snow guns were running non-stop. In the right room I could lay in bed and let the sound of the guns lull me to sleep. We were getting into *my* time of year. Each morning, I made a quick stop in the mountain parking lot to see what kind of progress they'd made the night before. I hoped they were doing as well at Gunstock.

I was supposed to work on Thanksgiving, but Dr. Rogers said, "Why don't you enjoy the holiday. This might be the last time for a long time that you won't be working them." I could have kissed the man. I went to my cousin Karen's for our annual gluttony event. Many of my relatives were there, and I fielded lots of questions about how I was doing. I found it surprising that I was no longer interested in talking non-stop about medicine. A year earlier, when I really didn't know anything, I happily offered an opinion on every health issue that came up. Instead, I sat at one end of the long dining room table and pursued an annual ritual: arguing with Karen's husband, John. We debated whether New Hampshire or Massachusetts had the more rational political system. I love to argue, but there's a problem in trying to argue with John: one minute he sounds like an ultra-conservative and the next minute like a dyed-in-the-wool liberal. I couldn't get a grip to really tee off on him. Afterwards we settled in to watch football games – over John's objections. He used to be a state trooper in Massachusetts. He'll watch reruns of any old cop show, even on Thanksgiving when there's football to be had.

All of a sudden my Uncle Pete, a man of ninety-something and still strong as a blacksmith, started to slide down on the couch. Karen, who'd been a nurse, noticed immediately and asked, "Dad, what's wrong?" Uncle Pete looked a little pale and sweaty. He said, "I'm having trouble breathing." My Aunt Therese said, "At least we have two medical people here." I was so shocked by the sudden event that I didn't feel like a medical people at all. My first inclination was to say to myself, "What the hell do I do?" I sat on the couch with him and rubbed his back. Karen went and called 911. I got my wits about me and took his pulse while asking him the basic questions about chest pain and nausea. He whispered, "No pain. Just pressure. I think I could throw up." Karen came back with a basin. We looked at each other. I said, "Get him an aspirin." Karen said, "He already had one today." I said, "I think he should have another one." She went upstairs. The siren of the ambulance whined in the distance. I hoped they were coming here.

They were. A paramedic and two EMTs came in the front door with an oxygen canister and a stretcher. They were matter-of-fact and joking as they went about their business. I stood out of their way. It felt odd that, for the first time in ages, I wasn't in the middle of something like this; it wasn't my place. This was their show. One of them asked Karen, "Do you want us to take him to Holy Hill?" That would be St. Elizabeth's, a Catholic hospital that sits on a rise on the outskirts of Boston. Karen had spent a lot of years there. She said, "Yeah. Let's go." Off they went, and it felt like they took a lot of the air in the room with them. The rest of us sat and stared at each other for a minute. Then Thanksgiving proceeded as planned, except for the several empty chairs during dessert.

It took the docs a few days to figure things out, but it turned out that Uncle Pete was having a severe bout of pulmonary hypertension. I'm pretty sure there wasn't a whole lot we could have done for him. I was really glad that Karen had been there. She'd taken charge.

Right after Thanksgiving we got our first major blast of winter. I awoke to a rip-roaring snow storm. I was driving from Gilford over to the hospital and figured I'd better allow an extra hour and a half, and it was a good thing I did. The snow was heavy and wet, and the driving was treacherous, even with all-wheel control. Stopping every five minutes to wipe the built-up snow off my windshield wipers, I made a mental note to get winter wipers at the earliest opportunity. At one point I'd considered calling the hospital and telling them I couldn't make it in. I'm glad I hadn't. I got there with about ten minutes to spare. As I pulled into the parking lot, the sun came out and started to go down at the same time. It sparkled off of the snow and ice in the trees and on the wires. I would have felt foolish not making it in. Besides, the emergency department is the last stop. You have to work. Along those lines, I once asked a doctor named George Shervanick if he ever considered himself too sick to go to work. Without a pause he said, "Nope. No matter how sick you are, you are in fact coming to a hospital. Get an I.V. in you. Get some fluids running and some anti nausea and anti diarrheal meds in you and you're good to go."

My clinical year ended on a bitterly cold day two weeks before Christmas. Dr. Rogers said, "I'm impressed with how far you've come. I now have no problem referring to you as a colleague." That was the absolute best compliment I'd gotten all year. I told him I was certain that I wanted to work in emergency medicine, and explained the role he'd played in that decision, going back to the time I'd chatted with him during the first year of school. His reply: "Just don't blame me if you don't like it or can't get a job."

On the ride home I thought about his comments. The liking it part was not an issue. I knew there was no other field that I wanted to be in. The getting a job part *was* a real concern. All you ever heard about in school and read about in articles was how PAs were in such demand. In fact, it was pegged as being one of the most in-demand careers for the next ten years. At the same time, no one had come running to offer me work. I knew several classmates who already had jobs lined up. They weren't in emergency medicine, though. They were all office-based or surgical. I found it interesting that of my twenty-two classmates, only one person was going to end up going into the area that he'd originally been interested in. A couple were now pointed at emergency. That made them competition for jobs. Still we all shared information about potential opportuni-ties. I had already started to follow the open position ads in the papers and on the internet. There were lots of jobs for PAs. Some were even in emergency medicine. The sobering side was that all of the emergency jobs required a minimum of two years experience. There were no offers of "we will train you" like you saw in other specialties. I decided not to worry right now. Graduation was a week away. The boards, which I had to pass to become certified and get a job, were a month off.

# Graduation

First things first. We all gathered at the school three days before graduation to try on our caps and gowns. The ritual of which side you wear your tassle on and the deal about having your sash presented and put on were explained. Some of my classmates would be receiving special honors; that was explained. We were told what time to be at the country club where the ceremony would be held, and to definitely not be late. We adjourned with everyone making plans to meet up for the class Christmas party the following evening, a chance for everyone to clean up, look their spiffiest and let their hair down.

The party was being held on December 15th, the night before graduation, in Concord, at a funky old hotel in a funky function room that took up most of the basement. A lot of the class would be staying at the hotel after the party. I decided not to. I was so much older than most of them that I felt like I'd be in the way. Also I didn't want to look hung over in my graduation pictures. This was the first chance to meet many of the spouses and significant others we'd heard so much about. I was by myself. Christy had her kids; she'd be coming the next day for graduation. I didn't mind. A big martini got me into a festive mood. The food was great. The women, including faculty, all looked stunning. It never ceased to amaze me that when you spend lots of time with people, they suddenly look so different when they're all glammed up. The band started and I was roped into several dances. I enjoyed every one of them. The hair was indeed coming down. It was great to see the other side of certain people. Julia Skladchikova, one of our Russian classmates, was probably the shyest person in the class, some of which was probably language- based, but she was definitely reserved. With a couple of shots of Stoli in her, however, she became the life of the party. She danced with total abandon, at times with a rose between her teeth, literally. The way she was shaking it, she would have fit in just fine at the old Whiskey A Go Go, dancing in a cage above the crowd. Her date was a big Russian guy dressed all in black. I said to Eric Horton, "Definitely KGB." He couldn't begin to keep up with Julia. I danced with Tracey Crossman, who was now several months pregnant. I told her I'd never danced a slow dance with a pregnant lady before. She gave a big laugh and someone took a pretty good picture of the two of us at that moment.

As the party really revved up, I decided to make my getaway before people got drunk enough to try and keep me from leaving. I said a few quick good-nights and walked out into a blast of cold air. The night sky was cloudless and the stars twinkled. While I was looking up admiring all that twinkling I almost fell on my ass, thanks to all the ice in the parking lot. I carefully picked my way to my truck.

Graduation day dawned with a major-league snowstorm. I decided to allow an extra hour to get to Manchester and the country club. I called first my dad and then Christy, both of whom assured me it was mostly rain in the Boston area. I had invited several family members, but because of the weather – and people being under the weather – it would just be my cousin Karen, my dad, and Christy. Christy and my dad were going to drive up together. That'd be interesting. There'd definitely be a fight over who'd do the driving.

Making sure I had my cap and gown, I got on the road. The driving was terrible – good thing I'd left extra time, all of which got eaten up because of a trucker who was having a hard time making it up a long hill, about two miles from the entrance to the Interstate. He backed down and tried again nine times. My windows were fogging up from the steam coming out of my ears. Finally a sand truck eased out into the other lane and made it up to the hill and laid down a huge swath of sand and salt. The trucker gunned it, his tractor trailer squirmed its way up and over, then he pulled off to the side of the road. Since I was now about to become a medical professional, I resisted giving him the finger as I drove past. I got onto Route 93 with a little time to spare – until I came upon three accidents in a row. Now I was traveling on borrowed time. I hit a stretch of road that wasn't plowed but I had to risk going faster than was comfortable. Then, as I got to Manchester, it dawned on me that I wasn't exactly sure where I was going. Nerves and the old tightness in my gut were setting in. I missed my exit while reading directions. I was going to be late. I came upon a toll booth and begged the attendant to make a quick directional switcheroo. She said, "Nope. Keep heading south for another ten miles. Then you can turn around." I started driving like a madman. I was going close to eighty in very bad conditions. I would have reported me to the state police. I figured that one of two things would happen if I got stopped: I'd either go to jail or get a police escort to the front door of graduation. Jail seemed the more probable outcome.

I found the country club and screeched into the parking lot where I saw Christy's car. Wow – she'd won the driving battle. I had no choice but to park quite a distance from the front door and got out swearing. I ran by Steve Cahill, still swearing. He yelled that he was just arriving too. I slowed down a bit, but kept swearing. My hair was soaked. We walked in together and found that the guests were just starting to enter the main room. Somewhere in the middle of all the people, Christy went up on her tiptoes and waved. She nudged my father who turned and nodded.

I rushed into the room where most of my classmates were already assembled in their caps and gowns. My little buddy, Cheryl, came running over and grabbed me. She looked worried. She said, "Calm down. You haven't missed anything." She helped me get into my graduation garb. Tracey Crossman told me, "Cheryl was so worried about you. It was cute." Yeah, real cute.

We got in line and marched down the hall, walking into a blast of heat in the overcrowded main room.. Finally I could start to relax! A flute and harp duo were playing something somber and all Pomp and Circumstancy. It was kind of emotional. I started to take it all in. I walked by the row where my father, Karen and Christy were sitting. They gave me big smiles, which added to the emotion. Honored guests, doctors and faculty were taking their places on the dais, wearing the various colored gowns, ribbons and big floppy velvet hats that serve absolutely no purpose outside of academia. Someone made a speech on the significance of the different colors of the robes and headgear, much of which had to do with being a part of the fraternity of medicine. The president of the college stepped to the front of the dais and said, "All rise to the graduating class of 2005." Next to me, Tracey Crossman burst into tears. I took out my handkerchief and gave it to her. She took a big, honking blow into it and started to return it. I said, "No problem. I don't really need that back." She giggled through her tears.

The speeches began. Our class president, Mark Barros, gave a wonderful speech. Tracey cried. The doctor who was our commencement speaker gave a wonderful speech. Tracey cried. One or two others gave wonderful speeches. Tracey was about cried out. I can't remember the content of most of the speeches, but they were all short and thus truly wonderful.

The time came to go up one by one for our diplomas. My name was called. I marched up there going a few rounds with my emotions. First, Louise Lee, the head of our faculty, put the sash of a graduate over my head and onto my shoulders. Louise is short and I am tall. I did a bit of an exaggerated back bend; there were chuckles in the crowd. I then turned and walked over to President Monahan, who held my diploma in his hands. I gave him an all-encompassing thank you and shook his hand. He said, "Now go out there and be a great PA." Returning to my seat, I drew a long breath.

Shortly thereafter, the flute and the harp started up again and it was time to march out. I was a physicians assistant. As I passed the row where my family stood clapping, I pointed to the ceiling and mouthed, "This was for you, Mom." Somewhere in the universe I had a very proud mother.

Everyone tumbled out into a large room set up with a bar and a full compliment of waitresses offering trays of hors d'oeuvres. Classmates milled about shaking hands with one another and introducing family all around. My first year advisor, Gale Furey, made her way over to where I was standing with my crowd. I introduced her to my family. She said, "I always enjoyed having Gerry around. He was a pretty good student." I said, "Dad, Gale is a pilot." My father had flown private planes for years; if the war hadn't robbed him of his left leg, he probably would have flown for one of the airlines or at least worked for them. They got into a long conversation about flying. I kept trying to steer the conversation back to the part about what a good student I was but they refused to come along. Gale had also just come back from maternity leave so we talked about her new son. Gale seemed to like flying even more than being a PA but, for her, flying wasn't going to pay the bills.

When I had done my internal medicine rotation at the VA hospital, I spent a day with her. She came in once a week to run a dermatology clinic. It was one of the best days I'd had in the rotation. Gale was as relaxed in the clinical environment as she'd been tough and such a stickler about everything in the school environment. She had me do all of the exams and then try to figure out what was going on. Skin is really hard to diagnose. I've seen more than one doctor walk out of an exam room and run for the dermatology atlas with all the pictures. Towards the end of the day, Gale had said, "Your next patient is a Carmelite nun." I said, "Huh?" Nuns and VA hospitals didn't seem to go together. Gale said, "She wasn't always a nun. During World War Two she flew bombers." I didn't know this, but apparently they'd used women to fly bombers from the factory to airstrips near the combat zones. They didn't fly actual missions but at times did find themselves flying in harm's way. I guess the government considered them more expendable than their combat-trained male counterparts. How times have changed.

The crowd was starting to thin as classmates and families began to leave. As I tried to pull my father away from Gale, I looked around and realized that I'd probably never see most of these people again. Funny, we'd all spent one year basically living together and now they were already starting to become strangers. We got outside and the cold air felt great. Christy was going to drive home with Karen, and I would drive my father home; we'd rendezvous in Waltham. The rain and snow had dampened down to a non-event. My father is not one to emote on anything. He did say on the ride home how impressive he'd found the ceremony and what a tremendous accomplishment this was for me.

We were headed to Waltham where I'd grown up and where he still lived, for a quiet family dinner at a little Italian restaurant in the center of town named The Chateau. I hadn't been there in a while. The Chateau wasn't so small anymore; business had been good. Walking across the parking lot reminded me of the scene in the Godfather when the bad guys pick Michael Corleone up for dinner in front of Dempsey's Restaurant. Neon signs reflected off icy pavement. I was pretty sure Lou Nocera, the owner, didn't let any bad guys in. I hadn't seen some of these aunts and uncles in almost a year. I really appreciated them joining us and enjoyed a relaxing and wonderful dinner.

On the ride to Christy's house we talked about the events of the day and who certain people were. She said, "I'm kind of surprised. You really weren't as emotional as I thought you'd be. You looked like you were just going through the motions." I replied, "I enjoyed it, but the real battle has just begun. I have to pass the boards and get a job." She asked, "Can't you just enjoy the moment?" I said, "Well, I'm bothered by something." She asked what that was. I said, "It really sank in during graduation how much older I am than the rest of the class. I'm wondering if people in the audience were wondering whose father was up there in the cap and gown. I felt embarrassed." She took my arm. She said, "Honey, all the more reason to be proud of what you've done. Besides, you're pretty well preserved. You didn't look all that much older than some of the class." Lovely girl.

Christmas of 2005 was a wonderful time. I was relaxed and enjoyed doing nothing. I was pretty sure that Christy's son was savvy to the whole Santa Claus routine and just went along with the status quo. On the other hand, her daughter was still a member of the Santa cult and with that went the sense of excitement, anticipation, and impatience that makes this a magical time of year. We'd all be better off if we were still members of the Santa cult.

The kid in me still likes to get a lot of stuff for Christmas. It doesn't have to be expensive but I love opening lots of packages. Christy understands this and so on Christmas morning, I had a pretty good pile under the tree with my name on it. Of all of my gifts, the one that meant the most was the long, white medical coat. It meant so much to me that she had thought to buy me one. I went over and gave her a big hug and a kiss that by kid standards was way too long. They both asked us to stop. Darn kids.

# Boards

My boards were scheduled for January 16, 2006. I spent most of my waking hours studying. The problem is that you can't go back and study two years' worth of learning in a couple of weeks; you'd make yourself nuts. This problem has been well addressed by books that serve as board refreshers, filled with the kinds of questions that you can count on finding on the exams. There are books out there specific to the PA boards but I couldn't find them and I was too lazy to go on line and order them. Instead I bought a couple of books for the medical boards that doctors take. I figured that if I could do all right with their questions, I could do all right with mine. I opened the first of these books to find question after question about stuff that I'd never heard of. This was *not* the way to start. I opened the other book. This contained material that looked a lot more familiar. Maybe this one was for dummy doctors but I didn't care. I needed to go into this exam with a sense of confidence. I tried to study a minimum of four hours a day.

That was tough. It required a lot of breaks to stare out the window. What I saw out the window was disheartening. After an early flash of winter, we went back to fall. No snow. No frozen lake. Yuck. Thank God for snowmaking.

When I wasn't studying, I was patrolling. One day as I rode up on the lift I thought, "Wow, man, you've come full circle." The seeds for my new career had been planted here and had now grown into something truly big. I could now look someone in the eye with pride and say, "I'm a physician assistant."

Very early one morning I walked into first aid base. Curt Golder had just gotten there and we had some time alone together. Curt now had the job of K-2, number two in command. Steve Brennan, who had left the patrol, had by chance met a wonderful girl who had been a fellow nursing student of mine. They'd bought a house and were now expecting a child. Steve decided it was time to earn an honest living and had gone to work in one of Wal-Mart's warehouses. Word coming back to the slopes was that he hated the real world. Pat McGonagle had divided Steve's job between Curt, Lee Bates and Kyle Davis. It was kind of like the corporate structure where you have vice presidents of operations, human resources, and marketing. In this case Curt was running day-to-day mountain operations, Lee was responsible for training and scheduling, and Kyle was responsible for investigating serious incidents and anything else that happened off mountain. I congratulated Curt on his new job. I told him I thought he had that special quality that made people want to work hard for him. He smiled and nodded his head in appreciation. He said, "I can't tell you how proud I am of you. Look where you came from and what you've become. I don't think many people could do that at our age."

We both brought up examples of some of my early missteps on the patrol. Curt kept rolling his eyes and doing an exaggerated dumb-slap of his shaved head as we recounted some of my first year. We laughed way too hard for this early in the morning. We talked about Kyle, who by chance had happened onto a series of accidents that were as serious as any we had ever dealt with, events that resulted in hospitalized skiers who still might die. She had handled each incident like a champ, but she was burned out by it. She said more than once, "I'd love to have a day where I can just ski and not find anyone." I had worked one of these with her; a skier had fallen out of the chairlift at the precipice at the top. He'd fallen a long way. Just getting in to the area where he was laying was exhausting. Kyle got there first and stabilized him. Ian Hamilton got there next and furthered the cause. If nothing else, Kyle knew she wasn't alone. I got there third with the help of one of the lift maintenance guys named Kevin, who brought me in on a four-wheeler, easily the scariest ride I've ever taken on the back of a vehicle. Each time we went airborne I yelled in alarm. He kept shouting back, "I'm sorry." I kept yelling in his ear, "Keep going." That ride was the most afraid he'd ever been at the mountain, he admitted to me later on. I was grateful I didn't know that while I was holding on to him for dear life. The injured skier was obviously hurt but still able to communicate with us pretty well. Later, given a full accounting of all his injuries, we all agreed it was amazing that he hadn't died in Kyle's arms. It was Pat McGonagle's day off but after a while, even he showed up on the scene. I guess he doesn't turn his scanner off too often. It was a tough extrication, most of which I spent sliding over icy rocks. I held the tail rope of the toboggan in my left hand and for most of the time, Pat's left leg in my right hand. He wasn't too thrilled about that.

January 16th came along and I was ready to kick ass. I drove to the testing center in Concord, tucked away behind a shopping mall, eventually finding it with time to spare. I sat in my car for a couple of minutes. It looked and felt like April. The middle of January and I wasn't even wearing a heavy coat. This global warming stinks. I went into the building, showed the guy at the desk the ninety-nine pieces of identification that were required and was directed to a cubicle. Its central piece of equipment was a computer terminal. The automated directions were tedious but clear; even I could understand them with no problem. I began taking the most important test of my life. It's funny that I can't remember how many questions there were – it wasn't that long ago. I think there were four hundred. I started at eight thirty and was done by about a quarter to one. I didn't find the test all that horrible. It was challenging, but most of the material covered was in areas that I should know. I walked out and called Christy. I said, "I think I passed." She was excited. I said, "Hold on. I *think* I passed. I don't know for sure." She replied, "There's no way you didn't pass." Her confidence level ranked considerably above mine.

The exam documents had clearly stated that it could take up to six weeks for the results to come back. They stated repeatedly that you should not badger the central office for your results. I took them at their word. I skied and patrolled – a lot.

One week later I was checking e-mails and found one that said, "Exam results." I went in six directions at once. I was sitting at the computer with my ski clothes half on and half off. One leg of long underwear was in a pile on the ground. I started tugging at the other leg. I couldn't get it off. If you can't get your underwear off, I was thinking to myself, how in the world can you expect to get your grade scores? I finally tore it off. I opened up the web site. It was requesting a password. Par for the course for me, I could not for the life of me remember my password. I called Christy, frantic. She said, "Calm down. Give me the website. We'll create a new password." We did. She opened the message. She read, mostly to herself but a little out loud. She was driving me nuts. All of a sudden she started audibly sucking in air. I kept shouting, "What? What?" She said, "You passed."

Two years of tension suddenly washed out of me in spasms of crying. I couldn't control myself. I cried for the best part of ten minutes. Please understand: I don't walk through life crying at the drop of a hat. It was the only appropriate response this time. Christy waited me out. Then we celebrated over the phone.

# Employment

Now it was time to go and get a job for real. I started to apply for every emergency job I came across. As I've mentioned, they all came with the caveat that two years of experience were needed just to be considered. I applied anyway. Sometimes a letter came back, usually from a doctor and generally stating how much they appreciated my applying but that they were pretty sure they'd stipulated a couple of years of experience as requirements for the job. Sometimes it was just a form-letter e-mail, the digital equivalent of , "Nobody with less than two years' experience need apply." Some hospitals sent nothing back; this surprised me. Even the worst toy companies always sent out letters in reply to inquiries about job opportunities. I guess that most hospitals considered themselves above most toy companies. They shouldn't.

I was getting frustrated. I decided maybe I needed to expand my horizons. I knew I wanted to work in a hospital environment, so I started applying for 'hospitalist' jobs, to be a PA responsible for patients once they'd already been admitted to the hospital. These jobs were asking for five years of experience. I was ready to give up and go for whatever job I could get. Christy kept saying, "Don't settle." Easy for her to say. It was March and I didn't have a nibble.

One day I was looking over the Internet job list. I saw a listing for an emergency room in Woonsocket, Rhode Island. Again, they wanted two years' experience So much for that. I didn't bother to answer.

One Saturday night Christy and I went out with the Dunfees. Tom Dunfee was a patroller with all sorts of advanced training. One night when I was brand new I'd been closing the top of the mountain. I thought I was doing a great job, but evidently he didn't agree. He jumped onto the radio and yelled, "Hey, you goddamned rookie, get it right." I'd sat back kind of bewildered and looked at Lee Bates. Lee said, "Tom must be having a bad day." I couldn't wait to meet him. One night I was working and he walked in. He was kind of a cool-looking guy. I walked up and introduced myself. His expression was one of distant recognition. I didn't mention the night that he had jumped on me. After working together for a few nights we started to connect. We had a lot in common. He and his wife were both sales reps. We could relate to the frustrations of dealing with national chains. His wife's name was Iliana (I think I got that right). She had an exotic look to match her exotic name, which was mentioned to Tom from time to time, at which he'd laugh and say, "Well, she's from Jersey City and I had to ask her father and five of her uncles for permission to marry her." He never said that it wasn't worth it. In the sixties Tom had been part of a rock band that opened for big time bands; he played lead guitar. As far as I was concerned, he was major league. He'd lived in Baltimore and opened for Nazz and Mott the Hoople. If the Beatles had been on his resume, I couldn't have been more impressed. He did all of the major Jersey Shore clubs. Iliana had followed him around. We got close. It turned out that one of his best friends was an emergency room doc who was engaged to a lady I'd once been involved with. His truly best friend was my doctor. I was afraid that the whole night would be a discussion about my personal foibles or my health.. Neither ever came up. Thank God for HIPPA. We had a couple of bottles of good wine at the Dunfee residence before we went out. Tom's guitars all sat in his study, cradled on metal racks, a collection of which Eric Clapton would have been proud. At dinner I sat catty-corner to Tom and talked guy stuff while Christy and Iliana sat cattycorner and talked girl stuff. I was pretty sure that the girls won out. We all made a pact to get together again.

On Monday, Christy and I got back to her house. I went back on line again. The job for the ER in Woonsocket, RI, was still posted. The part about two years of experience hadn't changed. I thought , "What the hell. It can't hurt to apply." I sent an e-mail, along the lines of "I don't have the experience that you're looking for. At the same time, having tons of real-life experience, I'm not your traditional student. If you believe that a strong work ethic and a desire to work emergency medicine are important, then you might want to give me a chance to talk." If frustration and anger can come through in an e-mail, it was present in what I sent.

A day later a message suddenly popped up on my e-mail. I sat stunned. I said, "Christy." She was talking on the phone. A little louder, I said, "Christy." She hung up the phone and walked over and said," What?" I opened the e-mail. It was from Daren Girard, as in Dr. Daren Girard. Christy started sucking in air real fast the way she does when she's excited. She started repeating real fast," Oh, my God. Oh, my God," which seemed pretty appropriate to me, too.

The letter from Dr. Girard said, "Hey. Got your e-mail. Interesting. We'd like to talk to you."

I answered it real fast. "Let's set a time."

I went in two days later for a meeting with a young-looking doc. I said, "Doctor, thank you for taking the time to meet with me" He said, "Please don't call me

'Doctor,' call me Daren." I told him I would, though, truth be known, I'm not comfortable calling doctors by their first name. If you couldn't tell from this book how much I respect doctors, then you must have skipped a few pages. No matter what they're like personally, they worked incredibly hard to become what they are and I feel they all should be addressed by title. Some people get a little too cavalier in making statements like, "Oh that crazy Daren," as opposed to," I talked to Dr. Girard." Call me old school.

However, I was prepared to call him Mahatma Ghandi if it would get me the job. I didn't have to. 'Daren' seemed to work pretty well. He introduced me to Paul Vallera, the PA in charge. He then took me down to the emergency department and introduced me around, announcing to each new person we came upon, "This is Gerry. He's a PA who'll probably be joining us." Man, that sounded great. He said of one of the nurses, "Don't get too close to Betty. She bites." I laughed. Betty bared her teeth and did a guttural Cat Woman growl.

We headed back to Dr. Girard's office. On the way he said, "I'd like to get you back in here to meet with Victor Pinkes. He's the Chair of the department." He asked, "How does two weeks from today work?" It worked. Tomorrow would have worked better.

On the ride home I was sky high. It felt like this job was mine for the taking. The fate angle wasn't too far outside my field of vision.

While waiting to get back for another meeting, I hopped to the process of getting licensed; I had to be licensed with the State of Rhode Island and the Federal Drug Enforcement Agency, and I had to apply for the job with Landmark Hospital. Each application involved piles of paperwork and supporting documentation. It also gave each place an opportunity to get into my wallet for anywhere from two to four hundred bucks. A scam wouldn't be too strong of a description of the process.

Evidently I passed my interview with Dr. Pinkes. The next day Dr. Girard sent an e-mail that said, "Welcome aboard. We'd like you to start on May 1." I was thrilled and relieved at the same time. I was coming to the end of one long road; another now lay directly in front of me.

Right before I was set to start, he called and pushed the start date to May 15. He said, "Enjoy this extended vacation. It will probably be your last one for a long time."

May 15 came good and fast. My first shift as a PA was to be from three in the afternoon to eleven at night. It seemed an odd shift to have for your first day but then medicine is renowned for not considering hours that the rest of the world typically lives by. After a workout in the basement, I paced around Christy's house for most of the day. The old nerves were building. At 1:45 I gathered up my brilliantly clean white coat, my stethoscope, and a couple of pens. I gave Christy a big hug. I patted Molly, Christy's one-year-old Pekingese, on the head. I've always gravitated towards big dogs but after spending time around Molly I think I'm won over. Christy calls her "my hairy little girlfriend."

I walked out the door and started the car. As I backed down the driveway I found myself thinking, "I wish I had another week before I started." As I drove up the Interstate towards Woonsocket, I thought, maybe they'll understand if I call in and say, "There's been a misunderstanding. I've change my mind. I don't want to do this." I kept driving. Eventually the hospital came in to sight. I parked across the street in front of a CVS drugstore, got out and walked towards a big sign that said Emergency. I leaned into a strong breeze, squinting against blowing sand. My white coat trailed behind me. Ambulances were parked out front in rows, like cars at the start of the Indy 500. I could feel the heat from their exhaust. I took a deep breath and walked up to a set of big, automatic doors. They slid open. I peered down the hallway, letting my eyes adjust. People in scrubs and long white coats were hurrying in all directions. Gurneys bearing patients of all ages and sizes were lined up against the walls. I stepped in. My real education was about to begin.

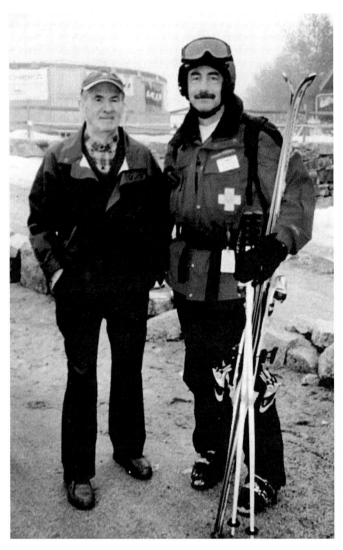

GERRY DOUGHERTY is currently working as a physician's assistant in a busy emergency room in Woonsocket, RI. His suturing has gotten a little bit better.

He splits his time between Gilford, NH, and Taunton, MA. He plans to continue to ski patrol at Gunstock as time and the management of Gunstock allow.